BIG KIDS

A Parents' Guide
To Weight Control
For Children

Dr. Gregory Alan Archer

Illustrations by Jay Walsh

Copyright © 1989
Gregory Alan Archer, Psy.D.

New Harbinger Publications, Inc.
5674 Shattuck Avenue
Oakland, CA 94609
All rights reserved
Printed in the United States of America

First printing January 1989 — 2,000 copies
Second Printing March 1989, 3,000 copies

This book is dedicated to my parents, Robert and Martha Archer, and to my grandparents, Clifford and Eleanor Archer. Without their support throughout college and graduate school, this book never would have been written.

I would like to thank Laine Walter, Ronald Kime, Ph.D., and Lorna Lemon for their critical review of the manuscript and helpful comments that moved a painfully rough draft toward the realm of readability. In addition, I would like to thank my literary agent, Martha Gore, for teaching me the way of books, and the staff at New Harbinger for their support and assistance in putting it all together.

Contents

Preface

Before entering elementary school, I was a happy-go-lucky kid, oblivious to the real world, doing the things most other five-year-olds did. By the time I entered first grade at Ledgeview Elementary, things had changed. Within a few days my classmates started to tease me, singling me out from the other kids because I was different — because I was overweight, or, more accurately, overfat.

I was a little overfat boy, an easy target for cruel jokes. Gradually, I withdrew into myself, pulling away from the boys and girls who should have been my friends. I remember the loneliness that marked my days at school.

As my weight continued to increase, so did the teasing:
Fatty, fatty, two by four,
Can't get through the bathroom door . . .

In the following years the bigger I became, the more insecure I felt. I wanted to escape. Hiding in the back of classrooms didn't work. One kid tossed paper wads at me for six months — I was hard to miss. So I studied hard, hoping to impress the class with my mind. That only resulted in a new taunt: "Teacher's pet."

When the class bully demanded, "Hey, fatso! Gim'me your lunch money. You sure don't need it!" I handed it over without a fight. I guess I didn't need it.

Television helped me to escape. Watching football gave me some solace; after all, those guys were big like me. Here was a place I could fit in. So when my few friends started a neighborhood game, I joined in the rough and tumble on the field. But when our sixth-grade classes started touch football teams, once again my weight became the target of ridicule: "Take a hike fat-boy! Nobody wants you on his team. Wait a minute, Archer could be the whole front line!"

Everyone laughed. But I did get on a team. And when the other boys saw how hard I tried, everyone wanted me on his side because "Archer could crush the other team." I played my heart out; I wanted to do something right.

Junior high school was a little easier. The coach, who knew my older brother had done well in sports, gave me a football uniform and a chance. I was elated and gave it my all so as not to disapoint him. Before long, I joined the wrestling and track teams, even though I was part of the "fat boys"—the upper weight classes. We even had a "fat-man's relay team" in track. I didn't care what they called it—I was in sports.

I was luckier than most overfat kids because, eventually, athletics showed me some of the secrets of weight control. My appearance improved and my confidence rose. I controlled my weight so well that my high school coaches told me I'd have to increase my weight to get a scholarship for football. I worked very hard. Unfortunately, in college my football career came to a sudden end. For once in my life I was too small.

Turning from sports to academics, I followed my mother's footsteps and studied to become a psychologist. In graduate school my thoughts returned to those unhappy days when I was an overfat kid. Those memories sparked my desire to know more about weight control. It soon became evident that one way to help was to show parents how their children could avoid the trials I had endured on the road to health and fitness. I began to research and develop a program to that end.

I have found that, given a supportive family and unpressured approach, most children can grow into their weight in a normal and natural process. By slowly changing eating habits to enhance enjoyment and to eat for the right reasons, by adding fun activities to family life, and by eating nutritious foods, most children can attain normal weight with time. The real key is to make it *fun* and make it a *family* effort.

Hence, my program was born. It's called Kid S.T.U.F.F. That's *System Training Using Family Fun.* The whole family learns ways of making weight control not seem like weight control. It *can* be fun!

Weight loss is a national obsession. A *USA Today* headline reads: "A third of girls are dieting, but most aren't fat" (5/3/88). This mass delusion cannot continue.

By changing habits early in life, you can help your family avoid the current nation pastime—DIETING. Dieting does not work and I will show you why in Chapter 1. And since eating disorders such as anorexia and bulimia are becoming epidemic, you can further help your kids to avoid psychological problems in the future by taking a reasonable stance on weight control now.

If we give our children the basic skills of weight control, they can avoid future weight problems and eating disorders. Food does not have to rule anyone's life. Don't let it rule your family.

Gregory Alan Archer, Psy.D.   4/19/88

Introduction

Anne started off loving school. But after being continually teased about her weight, she began to lose interest. Her parents didn't know what to do. Should they put her on a diet?

Shirley had been overweight as a child. She didn't want her daughter, Jill, to have the same problems. After trying for six weeks to get her to lose, Shirley gave up in utter frustration after Jill gained five pounds on a popular diet.

A history of heart disease ran through both Bill and Sandra's families. Bill's father died at age 54 from a heart attack. Their doctor said that their son, John, had high blood pressure and was overweight. The doctor recommended a diet. John was eleven.

Six-year-olds failing in school because of weight? Families fighting over eating? An overweight eleven-year-old with high blood pressure? It does happen.

Good intentions started our national obsession with weight. The original focus on health is good. However, the method of reliance on dieting is bad. And now some parents are allowing children to fall prey to the dieting monster.

At least 35 percent of the American population is overweight. Not included in the number is 16 percent of the adolescents and at least 11 percent of the elementary age children who are overfat. The number of overfat children has been steadily increasing since the 1960s. Since many parents have used diets for their own weight control, they are using dieting with their children.

Sound weight control is important. We know growing fat means running an emotional gauntlet and playing cardiac roulette. But many parents are too quick to see a problem.

For those children who are truly overfat, growing up is difficult emotionally. The teasing, the jokes, the attacks go on. Most overfat children suffer low self-esteem, reduced school satisfaction and impaired friendships. They often display a sense of failure and rejection.

As adults, overfat individuals continue to experience impaired relationships and poor self-understanding. School and job discrimination occurs. Fat adults receive lower pay in comparison with slim co-workers. Overfat people carry a continuous social stigma that is unnecessary and preventable.

Childhood overfatness very often sets the stage for physical disorders as well. Dr. Gerald Berenson of Louisiana State University found that obesity and high blood pressure in children contribute to heart disease later in life (*American Health Magazine*, January/February 1988). Studies on Korean and Vietnam casualties confirmed that soldiers as young as nineteen had signs of hardening of the arteries (artherosclerosis). It all began in childhood.

It is well recognized that the most severe forms of overfatness begin in childhood. If children don't control weight early in life, they may never do it. *Children who stay overfat throughout adolescence have only a one in ten chance of ever obtaining permanent weight control as adults.* Those are pretty poor odds.

It has been proposed that if we could eradicate overfatness and reduce associated disorders such as diabetes, high blood pressure and heart disease, the average life span would go up four years. Is that all that much? Contrast it to the fact that if *all* cancers were cured, life spans would only increase by two years.

But despite this, parents should not go overboard with weight control. Sometimes controls create more problems than solutions. Parents should not force children to diet. Kids should have free access to some foods but not others.

Parents should not force rigorous exercise. Kids should have lots of playtime and fun family games to engage in. Dieting alone cannot give long-term results.

You must understand that this is a book of weight control for children. Weight *control,* not weight *loss.* How are they different? Weight loss is what you get from a diet — a temporary measure to get rid of extra baggage. Shortly afterwards, however, most people find weight returns in endless cycles of ups and downs. The so-called rhythm method of girth control. It's unhealthy and destructive, especially for children.

On the other hand, weight control is the art and science of maintaining a healthy weight. It is a *process* rather than a temporary measure. We are not born with the knowledge of weight control. It takes conscious thought and effort, and training at an early age.

First, you will take a look inside your child's body and understand the physical aspects of overfatness. Next, you'll be looking inside your family and child's *mind.* You'll see how poor eating and exercise habits cause overfatness, and how psychological dynamics support and maintain overfatness. Once you have a good understanding of this complex picture of overfatness, I'll show you what you can do to reverse the weight gaining trends.

By first observing your family in everyday life, you will be able to find habits that need improvement. Once found, you can go about correcting those habits by teaching rules of weight control in a number of different ways. You will decide to try a particular technique. See if it works. If it does, then continue it — perhaps for a lifetime.

As you start reading this book, try to involve the whole family. You may want to sit down together and talk about it. Weight problems are a family matter. Search out ways of helping each other. Don't single out the overweight child as the person with the problem. Let the whole family reap the benefits.

Most of all, take your time and be consistent. Changes may be slow. Most importantly, you should not anticipate a large weight loss. *The ultimate goal is behavior change.* Do not be concerned with actual weight loss. For most children it is more important to *slow* down the rate of gain. This is a very different attitude than those applying to adult weight control.

One other caveat: *Overreacting to small or modest problems may actually increase the chances of the child becoming overfat or developing an eating disorder.* See this as a positive learning experience. Don't strive for perfection. Life is not perfect.

So, too, will you have to look at the way you approach food. Children learn by example. You'll need to set a good example.

To avoid problems, children need a healthy relationship with food. Let's see how your family may move toward a happier lifestyle by understanding overfatness and food.

Chapter One

The Stuff of Overfatness: What's Going on Here?

Overfatness is an excess of fat tissue on the body.

•

As long as more calories are taken in than the body can use, overfatness will occur. Rarely, however, will dieting alone "cure" overfatness.

•

Causes of overfatness are numerous. Often it comes from poor eating habits, getting too little exercise and eating for the wrong reasons.

•

At times, food is used to deal with emotions. Children must learn other ways to cope.

•

The consequences of overfatness are painful physically, emotionally and socially. Overfatness carries considerable social stigma.

•

Prevention is the key to success in avoiding lifelong problems. Positive eating and exercise habits must begin early to maintain weight control in later stages of life.

Anne was six years old. Her flaming red hair was usually drawn up into a pony tail. Freckles were sprinkled across her cherubic cheeks. She was apparently a happy child with many interests. Curiosity loomed in her eyes. She was fascinated by moving objects. She would spend hours watching things move, spellbound by action.

Her parents, Sandra and Dan, recognized that their child was quite remarkable. Evidence of intelligence puttered at their feet in the form of a child advanced beyond her years. Anne was accepted into a close and loving family and attention was lavished upon her.

She bloomed with gifts of thought and drawing. It was a natural feeling for her to take a pencil in hand and let it dance across paper. She spent hours mesmerized with creation. Her parents encouraged her explorations. With all the efforts expended on Anne, the rudimentary framework of a successful school career had been constructed even before she set foot in a classroom.

Then, as with all children who reach age six, a magical and scary moment arrived. Elementary school began. She set out to test her abilities in the classroom. Anne was eager to take the challenge as she jumped on the bus. She was off to Mrs. Thistleseat's First Grade.

From day one Anne loved school. She enjoyed the lessons, letters and writing which gave her the opportunity to show how much she knew already. Art, too, appealed to her. She spent as much time as she could learning different art forms.

Early on, her teacher recognized and commented on how intelligent Anne was. The early education put her beyond the average classmate. Her enthusiasm was special. Once a lesson was completed, she would be seen speeding on to the next subject. Quick to remember, quick to answer, Anne was a star pupil.

As the year progressed, however, Anne's interest at school began to wane. Dan and Sandra became concerned when grades started to drop. Something, and they weren't sure what, was affecting their daughter's performance.

Sitting down with Anne, they asked, "What's wrong?" Anne quickly looked away. Shoulders shrugged. "I don't know," was all she said.

Days later, Anne announced she wasn't feeling well. She stayed home. This happened three more times in two weeks. A pediatrician was consulted. An extensive examination resulted. The verdict? No physical problems were found. Unconvinced, the parents took her to another specialist. Again, no physical illness was diagnosed; but the doctor was a bit concerned about her weight. After more questions, Anne finally spoke. With pursed lips and teary eyes, she said she was mad at her classmates for calling her "fat."

Shirley had been overweight as a child. Recollections of being the brunt of jokes were still quite fresh in the back of her mind. She didn't want her daughter Jill to carry the same past. When a few bulges appeared on Jill, Shirley became quite concerned.

Objectively, Jill, eight years old, was mildly overfat. She had a few ripples and bulges here and there, and a slightly curved paunch preceded her steps. Alternatively, her roundish face displayed pep and vigor. She appeared healthy and she was rather active.

Shirley decided that Jill needed to lose weight—immediately. First, Shirley started to restrict the amount that Jill was to eat. That decision did not go over too well with Jill. As she was a healthy, growing child, hunger came often. Between meals, Jill would get into cookies or potato chips or candy. Shirley knew it is common, and even necessary, for children to snack. But as the bathroom scale inched upward, Shirley decided to stop the nibbling. Not unexpectedly, Jill protested quite loudly—loudly enough that, eventually, pitched battles erupted.

One after another, skirmishes flared and the warring parties took up sides. Each tried to hold on to their snacking position. The war zone eventually overflowed onto the dinner table as Shirley then tried to cut Jill off from table foods. Jill, filled with anger and resentment, tried to eat more.

During an escalating incident, Jill's hands darted back and forth to the dishes on the table. Shirley, growing tired of the antics, slapped Jill's knuckles. Taking spoon in hand, Jill loaded it with vegetables, turned and fired. With peas rolling off her shoulder, Shirley was not amused.

In the meantime, across the table, Shirley's husband, Dave, was exasperated with all the jousting. His eyes shifted back and forth. He did not know who to be most angry with that day. In part, he was angry with Jill for not doing what her mother was saying. On the other hand, he felt Shirley was unreasonable at times. He did not interfere for fear of making things worse. Caught in the middle, not knowing what to say, Dave retreated into frustration and anger. What could he do?

Jimmy's baby pictures were of a rather plump little guy. His eyes were tucked back in a roundish, pink face. A wisp of hair fell by his left ear. His arms and legs were thickly segmented. He came into the world at eleven pounds, three ounces—a bit heavier than the average baby. (His mother had known that through her 23 hours of labor!) Jimmy had been born to Susan and Bill. Since Jimmy's reluctant entrance, they had had one other child, John.

The family was middle class and Midwestern—a strong combination of the work ethic and firm beliefs in country. Hard work was reflected in the calluses on Bill's hands. His trade was construction and Susan worked beside him as a clerk in the contracting office. Though hard work was plentiful, money was not. Simply enjoyments were important. They would reward themselves after a hard day's work. Meals were a big portion of that reward.

Susan and Bill were brought up on meat and potatoes. It was a meal born of hard work. They grew up on meat and potatoes; their parents grew up on meat and potatoes. Work required food. Their understanding of food was red meat flanked by enormous spuds.

Susan always searched for the best she could afford. She hunted down the best potatoes and prime cuts of beef. To make dinners special, mounds of sour cream and butter carefully crowned the potatoes. The beef was broiled to perfection. What's more, she always prepared more than the family could possibly eat. Anything short of this daily feast meant to her that she was not fulfilling her duties as mother and wife.

In the evenings, Bill ate with abandon. All that lifting and nailing and pulling and gluing required sustenance. "Real" food was needed to drive all that activity. He layered his plate with anything and everything and never left a crumb. Seeing his father, Jimmy raced to eat heavily in turn. John followed in a close second. Finishing up, the boys vacuumed their plates so no stray morsel could make a getaway. Bill took pride in how the kids followed in his wake. "Like father, like sons," he thought. The boys were learning how to eat like Dad, how to eat like "men."

Eating "like Dad" was very flattering to Bill. Unfortunately, Jimmy wasn't getting nearly the exercise his father was, and all the eating was causing him to balloon in size. John, too, wasn't far behind.

Bill didn't see a problem, but Susan did. She first noticed in an indirect, roundabout way—because of the household costs. The boys were growing out of their clothes faster than the budget would allow. Not just growing taller as most children do, but growing sideways, spilling tummies over belts, making pants unwearable. Moreover, food bills were skyrocketing but the cupboards were often bare. What could they do to stop the kids from excessive weight gain, as well as to avoid going broke?

What these three families have in common is that they are drifting toward overfatness. Some family weight problems are obvious: eating too much. Some family weight problems are complex: being caught in a power struggle over who determines how much and what can be eaten. Regardless of the type of problem, most families can find solutions. Each solution is unique and can be achieved by different pathways.

Throughout the chapters, you will follow these families in their quest to find weight control. Each family has its common strengths and weaknesses, and discover specific tactics for weight control. Those tactics can be used in any way that is best suited to your family.

With consistent effort and direction, you can help your family control weight in a reasonable way—no extreme changes, no ridiculous diets. No need to consider a complete swearing off of "fattening" foods, either. Your family changes habits to eat reasonably, exercise regularly and choose foods rationally. Ultimately, together you build personalized lifetime control, rather than gamble on a short-term fix.

Using common sense advice, weight control is a normal, natural process. All average weight people have learned to take control in their own way. Your family will find its own special way to take control. Any bad habit can be changed. It is a matter of learning and a matter of unlearning. You may find only a few eating and exercise habits need to be unlearned. Or maybe you will choose to make many changes. The choice is yours.

It has long been recognized that bad eating and exercise habits are difficult to break. Change becomes harder the longer the problems remain. The more "practice" that goes into learning patterns, the more effort is needed to break them. This is why most overfat children grow into overfat adults: Too much effort is required to break too many habits. It is best to prevent overfatness in the first place. But what is overfatness?

Overfatness

Overfatness exists when the amount of fat, known as adipose tissue, is excessive. The real trick, however, is judging what *is* excessive.

There are a few easy techniques to use as a guide to determining whether your child is overfat. The eyeball test is usually reliable. Look at your child and see if he is in good proportion. A little bulge at the waist? Not to worry. Only if the child's waist measurement is much more than the chest measurement do you have a direct indicator of overfatness. A stocky build is not a problem. A large bulge at the waist could be.

A second technique is the ruler test. Start by having the child lie on his back. Place a ruler lengthwise from the stomach to the chest. If the ruler does not lie flat, too much fat is being carried at his belly.

Above all, if you have questions as to whether your child is overfat, and by how much, talk to your pediatrician. He or she can do more sophisticated testing if necessary.

What About Normal Growth?

Before we launch into what causes overfatness, we must know what normal is. Normal growth patterns in children follow a predictable course. Generally, infants rapidly increase in body weight from birth to approximately five months of age. They gain about 20 grams (¾ oz.) per day during this period. At five months, the gain decreases to 15 grams (½ oz.) per day for the rest of the first year. At that rate, the infant will double its birth weight in the first five months and triple it in the first year.

During the second year the body continues its rapid growth. The infant will gain 5–6 kilograms (12 lbs.) in weight and nearly 12 centimeters (5 in.) in height. In addition, growth becomes more variable for each child. Weight gain may come quickly at one time and more slowly at another.

Usually, the perfectly average five-year-old is about 43 pounds, and the normal range is between 32 and 52 pounds. Both boys and girls in this age group grow in a fairly identical fashion.

Shortly before entering adolescence, male and female growth patterns split from a parallel path. The growth spurt begins for girls at age 10 and 11 and for boys at age 12 to 13. Soon afterwards, a rash of changes occurs.

Physical maturation comes in bursts. Adolescents gain and lose weight. Height skyrockets. Fat levels change. Girls become women. Boys become men. Parents become anxious. After this hormonal riot, they settle at or near what should be their full adult weight.

The spurts end at age 17 for women and age 19 for men. Essentially, growth has ended. In the next few years a few more pounds are added as muscle tissue matures. But physiologically, there is no reason to ever be heavier later in life. That's right, no reason to weigh more. What did you weigh at 21?

If variability is normal for kids, how do you know if your child is growing normally? Your pediatrician can know for sure. Most physicians can readily identify any significant deviations out of the growth curve. Most often, gains or losses are really nothing to worry about. Children reacting to stress or physiological changes will often demonstrate fluctuating weight. However, if your child has had considerable rapid gains or losses, see your doctor.

Normal Eating Habits

Being a parent, you may have discovered that the words "normal" eating habits and children should not be used in the same sentence. All children's eating habits vary widely. So what is normal?

Eating can be as variable as growth patterns. Strange habits tend to arise spontaneously. Such behaviors stress the parent more than the child. Knowing that normal kids eat in highly unusual and idiosyncratic ways can help you to understand that just letting it happen *at times* is acceptable. Childhood can be a little crazy. That's the fun of being a kid. Don't get upset if he likes peanut butter on a hamburger.

As children pass from the explosive growth of infancy, they become more discriminating in tastes. They like to pick and choose, to exercise independence at home. Parents have a tough time here, because as the child's growth varies, hunger drops off. Eating becomes erratic. Parents worry if the child is eating enough. For instance, between the second and third years, weight can drop for no particular reason — growth may have slowed so hunger diminishes. Weeks can pass without much growth or enthusiasm for eating. Periods of "don't want nothin'" crop up. These times are normal.

Within this time of scattered eating habits, some children decide they are only going to eat what *they* want to eat. At a particular moment, that may be a single item. Parents become aggravated attempting to get a child to eat more. This is part of learning effective interaction and control: finding out what they can and cannot do. So don't be overly concerned or force him to eat other foods. Kids want to learn independence and control their world. It is a learning phase children go through. Most resistance will pass with time and patience.

Playing with food can become part of that resistance. Again, don't be too concerned. Don't demand perfect etiquette, but have reasonable expectations for what should happen at the table. Let the children feel some degree of control. Let them learn how to make choices at home so competent choices can be made elsewhere. After all, parenting boils down to teaching children to do for themselves.

Recognize that all children display resistance in one form or another. It is not that they set out to defy you directly. It is an expression of desire for mastery of themselves even though they lack the skills for higher levels of control. They want to do for themselves.

When children start school, cafeteria lunches give further independence in the food-choice arena. Now the child can pack a lunch or eat what is offered by the lunchroom staff.

As the child has been growing, the same nutritional needs are present as in past years, only greater quantities are necessary. The child must pick and choose to meet increased caloric demands. Strong peer influences shape new tastes. Bizarre childhood delights from potato chip sandwiches to Mexican nacho chocolate chip cookies can be spawned by the prodding of friends. That's the fun of being young—you'll try anything . . . once.

Essentially, it comes back to this: "NORMAL" EATING HABITS DO NOT EXIST. Each and every child can and will be different to some degree. Children need time to explore food and drink. Tastes wax and wane. They change so fast, parents must try to provide some support for the child's desires while holding to *some* limits. Parents must also be a model of good eating behavior. How to do that comes later.

Why Are They Overfat?

The formula for balanced weight is *calories eaten = calories expended for exercise or movement plus calories to maintain body.*

A calorie is the basic unit of food energy. It is to food as the gallon is to gasoline: a common unit of measure. If Billie lays down for 40 seconds, he will burn one calorie. Reading or sitting takes about two calories per minute. Running with his dog uses about 13 calories per minute.

When the number of calories eaten is more than the number burned, the body stores the remainder as fat tissue. Weight is gained. To gain one pound of fat, you must eat an extra 3,500 calories. To lose one pound of fat, you must *burn* an extra 3,500 calories. *No other way exists for losing weight.*

No matter what anybody claims to the contrary, calories have to be burned to lose weight. Some "authorities" claim that by eating certain foods or combinations you can lose weight. Hogwash! Actually, as you grow tired of eating the same prescribed foods every day, you naturally begin to eat less. As you eat less, you get fewer calories. It's weight loss through boredom, not magic.

Since you are bored, you can't keep eating in the same manner for long. The weight you just lost, and more, comes back as the old habits surface. And since metabolism has been slowed by the diet, weight piles up faster than before. Calories do count.

Further, a calorie is a calorie is a calorie. In other words, it does not matter where calories come from. If it's more than your body needs, you gain weight. If you eat too much of anything, you can become overfat.

All calories are used to power motion and exercise. Calories stoke the "cellular furnaces" to make muscles move. They are broken down in a very complex procedure. The breakdown releases energy which is captured by the cell for work.

Some research shows that most overfat children do not get enough exercise or expend enough energy. Studies on overfat adolescents showed that they vastly overestimated the amount of exercise they were doing. Because many children are bored by "exercise," they need to engage in fun activities to burn more calories. Fun games and activities are *the* most important way to control weight.

Continuing with our balanced weight formula, the second half of the equation shows where the rest of the calories go: *maintenance of the body.*

The number of calories used for bodily functions other than movement is known as the Basal Metabolic Rate, or BMR. The BMR includes the number of calories used to run the brain, digestive system and all other organs. People vary in calories needed for their BMRs. The variance is due to different levels of muscle tissue, efficiency of organs and some poorly understood processes. (We believe the differences in BMR may be the reason some people have a tough time losing weight.)

In addition, repair of tissue requires a great deal of resources. Food, especially protein, is broken into its basic parts and used as building blocks for cells. Despite the large calorie requirements of maintenance and movement, it is still easy to get too many calories. When more calories are available than are needed in these systems, the body cannot dump all the extra calories. Once a calorie has been absorbed into the bloodstream, if it is not used, it is stored as fat tissue.

Fat, in and of itself, is not bad. In fact, life would not be possible without it. It performs many vital functions. Most of all, it stores calories for emergencies when considerable energy is needed. If you get caught without food, your bodyfat can keep you alive for days or weeks (some longer than others). It is a gold mine of energy at nine calories per gram. Carbohydrates and proteins only supply four calories per gram. Fats are also basic and necessary in nutrition. They are used in body processes and assist in the transport of vitamins. Only when fat is excessive does a problem surface.

Physical Causes of Overfatness

Oftentimes, parents believe that a medical problem is responsible for their children's overfatness. The truth is, however, physical problems are at fault in only about 3 percent to 5 percent of *all* cases. Endocrine disorders and genetic defects are quite uncommon. Medical tests can rule them out. If you have any doubts about your child's medical condition, see your pediatrician.

Physical factors can play a part in overfatness. Genetic traits will determine physical growth. Knowing the family history, we can predict how many children can become overfat. For instance, Johnny has only a 10 percent chance of becoming overfat because neither parent is heavy. Sally has a 50 percent chance because her father is overfat and Bill has an 80 percent chance because both his parents are overfat. This risk comes from a mixture of heredity and learning.

To understand the genetic link, scientists examined sets of twins. As could be expected, twins are very similar to each other in amount of bodyfat. Identical twins, who share the same genetic code, were extremely close in weight. If one was overfat, so was the other.

A number of the twins were placed in different homes at birth. Since the children lived in separate homes, they were subject to different eating rules. If their weights were still very similar, learning can't be the sole cause for overfatness.

This is the case. Most twins were very close in body-weight. This seems to support the notion that the genes we inherit from our parents impact on the development of over-fatness. Body structure, to a great degree, is handed down from one generation to the next. Hard work alone cannot guarantee a perfect body.

Although some children *are* predisposed to overfatness, that does not mean that a child *will* be overfat. It would be easier for overfatness to arise in children of overfat parents if poor eating and exercise habits are part of the family's makeup. Conversely, the child with very slim parents might have to eat more and exercise even less to become overfat. Under the right circumstances, however, anyone can become overfat.

What Does It All Mean?

Many theories have been proposed over the years about why overfatness occurs. Three of the most current examine the physical onset of overfatness. Basically, they address the physical evolution of adipose tissue, independent of other factors. These are the **fat cell theory**, the **sluggish metabolism theory** and the **set point theory**.

The fat cell theory states that people who are overfat may have an excess of fat cells in their bodies. Studies show the average adult has around 20 to 30 *billion* fat cells. In the first year of life, the number of fat cells increases six-fold. Infants are born with three to five billion. The cells continue to divide in the first few years until their numbers reach a little below the 20-billion level.

Normally, the number of fat cells stays fairly constant until adolescence. A few million cells are gained here and there, year by year. Males then increase fat stores during ages 11 to 13. A short time later, continuing hormonal altera-tions associated with puberty cause fat to be redistributed. Muscle tissue increases and the relative amount of fat di-minishes. Any remaining excess "baby fat" is *supposed* to disappear. The number of fat cells stabilizes around the 20-billion level in the average man.

In women, fat cell growth appears more varied. Females accrue fat cells during alternating periods. Between ages eight to 13 years are prime times to increase the fat cell number. Adding a few billion is normal. That's when it begins to get easier to tell the girls from the boys. The X chromosome signals the female's body to stock up on extra adipose tissue in preparation for child bearing.

As girls wander through puberty, changes become more pronounced. Hormones cause an increase in hip and breast density. The chromosomal and hormonal influences cause women to end up with more body fat. Less muscle tissue is developed in comparison to males. Adult men average about 15 percent bodyfat, while women average about 23 percent bodyfat.

The fat cell theory simply states that overfat people have gained too many cells at critical growth periods. The extra cells were gained in times of overfeeding in childhood and adolescence. So what? Well, an overabundance of cells can be a problem. All these extra fat cells work to keep themselves full.

An overfat person may have three to four times the number of fat cells than the average weight person — as much as 60 to 80 billion fat cells. Match that with the fact that each single cell has the capacity to expand two to three times its original size. The result is a tremendous storage capacity. The crowning blow is that once the cell is created it exists for life. You really cannot decrease the number of cells once they are formed. The overfat person is a walking lipid reservoir. An impaired ability to lose weight is the result.

The theory states that since cells naturally function to stay full, a person who gained weight at the critical times is likely to have more trouble controlling weight. A cell is developed to perform a function. It works to do what it is programmed to do, just like a computer. If the function is blocked and not fulfilled, the body reacts in some adverse way.

In part, this imbalance appears as hunger. As diets progress, the cells start to give up their fat cargo. Eventually, a majority of these cells are at low levels of lipids. A mechanism which is not well understood sends out a chemical message of "I'm hungry." Thus, the person is activated to feel hungry, even though he doesn't need food.

With the conflict between the dieter's desire to lose weight and the cells craving more lipids, feeling better physically hinges on being at a heavier weight. After fighting the feelings of hunger for many days or weeks, our embattled dieter may give in to the urge and eat more.

In addition to just eating more, since the cells are crying "starvation," the BMR has already slowed to use fewer calories. The leftover calories that would have been used to maintain the body are now stored as fat. Thus, even if eating is minimal, weight is gained back. Attempts at losing weight are thwarted by the body's own anti-starvation defenses. The person stays overfat despite well-placed efforts and intentions.

The second physiological theory proposes the "sluggish metabolism." It states that overfat people may need fewer calories to exist. Their BMRs are slower. Basically, overfat people require less energy to keep their bodies going.

Adipose tissue requires very few calories to maintain. Muscle, on the other hand, requires many more. This fact impacts on overfat people who have lost muscle through dieting or lack of exercise. Even if overfat people eat an "average" amount, some calories can be stored as fat because fewer calories are necessary for living. Therefore, a muscular 150-pound person could eat more and not gain weight, as compared with the overfat 150-pound person.

Greater muscle mass is one reason why men can eat more than women. Since men naturally have more muscle, they need extra calories for maintenance. Men have a natural advantage in weight control because of muscle. And since they weigh more on the average, every pound needs calories for upkeep; another reason men can eat more. (I know it's not fair!)

The sluggish metabolism theory is the weakest of the three theories because recent research shows that in a comparison of overfat people, data did not necessarily show them to have a consistently lower BMR, or daily caloric output. In fact, overfat people can use a considerable amount of calories in basic movement. This comes down to the laws of physics. Moving a heavier body takes more energy than moving a lighter one.

The theory does further highlight how the BMR reacts more efficiently each time a person goes on a diet. As caloric intake decreases, the BMR goes down. Subsequent diets make the BMRs downward spiral occur more and more quickly. Diets fool the body into thinking it is starving.

When we were living in caves, the decreasing BMR saved our lives when food was scarce. Now that we have an ample food supply, we don't normally need a survival mechanism. The body doesn't know that though. When we "starve" ourselves with restrictive diets, the body gets into a panic. All unnecessary activity shuts down. Thus, even if you eat very little, your weight loss slows. Eventually the diet stops working altogether.

The human body had about a million years to evolve survival tactics. Any perceived threat will be fended off—diet or illness alike. That's why diets don't work.

Our third theory is the set point theory. The main concept here is that people have a unique weight at which their bodies feel "comfortable." Normally, adults of *average* size will stay within 10 to 20 pounds of a specific weight. The ideal weight that the body fluctuates around is known as the "set point." The bathroom scale normally fluctuates on a daily basis (that's why you shouldn't weight yourself everyday), but overall weight stays near an average point.

The process is similar to a control on a furnace. You set a control for a specific temperature and the furnace will keep the house right around that temperature. When the room gets too cold, the furnace comes on; when too hot, it goes off. The body works in the same way. Weight centers around the set point and if weight gets too high or too low, the body compensates.

Some interesting research showed that when *average* weight *adults* were forced to eat excessively, after putting on about 20 pounds, it was harder and harder to keep gaining. Some people just stopped gaining all together despite large intakes of calories. (Remember, these were people who never had weight problems in their lives.) It was as though the body's weight thermostat turned off and pounds couldn't be added. The body initially resists going beyond a comfortable point even when eating continues.

What is happening to all those extra calories? You know that when the fat cells are depleted or empty, the BMR drops. That makes weight harder to lose because of decreased caloric need. When you eat too much, on the other hand, the BMR appears to increase to use up part of the excess. If the fat cells are full, storage ceases temporarily.

When our storage capacity is at its maximum, calories may not be absorbed efficiently. Some merely pass out of the intestinal tract. The body can't keep what it can't store. It appears that only after continuous, heavy overeating will more fat cells develop in the average weight adult.

Taking the example further: If the body did not regulate itself in some way, the world would have many more overfat people. And many of the overfat individuals would be much larger than they are now. If Samuel exceeded his caloric needs by only 4 percent per day, say 60 calories — one extra pork sausage at breakfast — he would gain 6 pounds in a year. If he continued to eat that extra sausage for ten years, he would gain 60 pounds. His bodyweight has risen from 160 pounds to 220 pounds. In ten more years, that sausage has put Sam at 280 pounds. Gaining 120 pounds in twenty years? Clearly, most adults do not fall into this trap. The body compensates for minor overindulgences.

According to the set point theory, if the body's set point is 160 pounds and the person weighs 180 pounds, extra calories would be excreted or burned in an attempt to stay near 160 pounds. Being heavier than the set point causes loss of excess calories. The farther away weight drifts, the harder and harder it is to gain.

Alternatively, if overeating made the set point high (220 lbs.), and the person now weighs 180 pounds, any extra calories will be absorbed. Absorption of calories will continue until he reaches the set point. The body will "fight" to get closer to 220 pounds by slowing BMR and gathering all excess energy for storage.

It seems that activity and exercise is the only way to modify the set point. Children can obtain lower set points by engaging in fun activities and exercise. Growth likely keeps the set point flexible. Exercise, as is explained in Chapter Four, will keep your child flexible.

So what we know thus far is that heredity influences overfatness. But this still does not really answer many questions. Research into the non-physical causes of overfatness suggests there is more to it than eating too much and fighting with hungry cells. We find that without certain conditions being met, a child will *not* become overfat. What are the other conditions?

The Family

Tony was the youngest member of a large Italian family. Since before he was born, food was a family affair. It was included in any sort of get-together, occasion or holiday. This was the tradition.

Once started on solid food, Tony was encouraged to eat as much as he wanted. His parents, Enrique and Maria, were big people and they wanted a "healthy" son. Food was a way of assuring health. Tony blossomed in that respect. He gained weight. For years the trend lingered on. He continued to grow bigger and looked older than his nine years.

Upon entering a new school system, he was noticeably one of the largest children in fourth grade. He stood out in a crowd of children. He stood out in his class so much that the school nurse was concerned. He fell in the uppermost percentages of the growth charts.

Tony's family turned out to be an especially good case study because his family illustrated a number of *overfat traits*. These traits are patterns of kindred behavior that produce and support an overfat life style.

The first pattern is culturally based. Some ethnic groups place heavy emphasis on eating. As with Tony's family, it is a sign of respect to the cook and family that you eat what had been prepared. The cook felt insulted if you did not eat. Everyone ate, regardless of hunger. Further, food was a sign of affection. Cakes, pies or treats were given to show how much you cared. It was love in a pastry shell—sugar as kinship. Finally, food was a reward at every occasion. "Sit down, eat!" and "Here, have a snack," was often heard. Food had taken on multiple roles that permeated social interaction.

Meals were a social event and all were expected to fill their mouths—often to excess. Tony's family was a prime example. Get-togethers occurred on most weekends. Food consumption was the main activity. There wasn't much else to do. No other activities were encouraged. The entire family engaged in too little activity to burn off too many calories.

Enrique and Maria prepared a great deal of pasta. It was the number one staple in the pantry. Unknowingly to them, the family's food selections had been mostly restricted to starches. They knew pasta was satisfying and stuck with it. Little else crossed the table. All were reluctant to try lower calorie selections. Tony was just as reluctant.

The restricted menu contributed to family members becoming overfat. Additionally, as Enrique and Maria were already rather large, Tony had the physical traits for overfatness. Since the life style was one of unrestrained eating, high calorie foods and little exercise, Tony was slated to become overfat. Some changes in habits had to occur or the health of each and every family member was at stake.

Armed with that knowledge, here is what Tony's family did.

First of all, the parents tried new foods. New dishes were introduced with fanfare and anticipation. Everyone was encouraged to sample the new cuisine. The parents took the initiative to begin to dig in. Tony was encouraged, not forced or bribed, to eat. Slowly, a few morsels made it to his mouth. Eventually, he ate some lower calorie foods but still felt full and satisfied. As before, the family ate many of the old standbys, but in moderation.

The next step was to target the eating style of the family. Families have specific rules that guide table behavior. Tony's family was observed to eat very fast. They did not pause very often; it was fork to mouth almost constantly. Since they ate so fast they really did not pay attention to what was on the plate. Enjoyment suffered. You can't enjoy a tidbit that never brushes the taste buds.

Eating slower made them more apt to feel full by eating less. By focusing on the food and trying to taste each bite, the food seemed more flavorful. It was more satisfying. As they knew how much was eaten, periodic pauses helped them to concentrate on how full they were. Once they were full, more often than not, they put down the forks.

Also, specific practices were employed to decrease the noise and activity at the table. Everybody was doing everything, every which way. At times, it was like yelling "fire" in a movie theatre.

Tony's parents tried to direct things a little more by having topics for discussion. Topics revolved around school, work, family, the universe. The communication led to closeness and a more pleasant atmosphere. Now they were learning how to truly enjoy eating by slowing down and feeling relaxed at the same time. As they settled into a pattern of enjoyment, the family began to consume less.

Despite the positive changes that were occurring, Tony still needed some limits. Prior to the program, he could eat anything and as much as he wanted. That much freedom of choice is not appropriate for children of his age. Enrique and Maria began to decrease the *types* of high calorie foods he ate by changing what was in the refrigerator.

He could eat as much as he liked of certain foods. The parents put no limits on such things as fruit and vegetables. Tony could have as much as he wanted, anytime he wanted it. Alternatively, cake, ice cream, junk food, etc. had to be limited—but not eliminated. Once a week or so it was OK to have a little junk snack. After a month or two, Tony began to eat many more vegetables than before.

At another point, a remake of the family reward system was necessary. Previously, Tony was given candy when he did well in school or did his chores. Substitution of fruit for a reward helped Tony to eat better. Most often he would get fruit, but some candy was still available—once in a while. Similarly, if Tony hurt himself, Maria would be too willing to use treats as a way of helping him feel better. Attention and hugs replaced those treats. A hug meant so much more. Tony readily accepted this.

Finally, Tony was not getting enough exercise. At school he was as active as most of his friends. At home he did very little. Watching television was his main pastime. He played outside about one hour for every four hours of watching TV.

Tony's family was not prone to exercise. Erroneous ideas colored their thinking about exercise. They thought it was "too much work" and "boring." Anything short of dashing down the street, huffing and puffing, knees ready to buckle, was not exercise. After playing some games that were fun but vigorous, the family came to recognize that exercise could be, heaven forbid, enjoyable.

The family members agreed to engage in activities a few days a week, but mostly on the weekends because the parents worked. Playing games naturally increased their time spent in exercise. When games didn't tickle the family fancy, an acceptable alternative was taking the dog for a walk at night. Twenty minutes was all that was needed. Exercise *was* like-able, and was done every day without disrupting the family's evenings.

Some other alternatives for increasing exercise were discovered. The car stayed in the garage more often. Walking to the store, walking to friends' homes and walking to school replaced driving. Tony and other children from his area got together to go to school. It was fun and a good way to make friends.

Little things began to add up. The whole family was burning more calories and taking in less. With just a little more effort, the calories used up everyday made a difference. This new life style caused some important improvements for Tony. His weight gain was slowing even though he was a rapidly growing young man. Noticing that difference kept the family moving.

Tony's weight eventually peaked. As he grew, fat began losing its hold on his body. Proportionally, he was looking much more like an average guy. He appeared happier and healthier. The entire family was healthier. They had met their number one goal.

You have just had a quick glance at one family's complete Kid S.T.U.F.F. Program. Your program may or may not be as extensive as theirs. It is up to you.

What are two or three problem areas that you share with Tony's family?

1. _____
2. _____
3. _____

Tony's family had a number of specific problems that tended to be easy to identify. But problems can be more subtle. Consider Shirley and her daughter Jill. They were presented as the second case in the beginning of the chapter.

From an outside vantage point, it was not difficult to see that the two of them were caught in a power struggle over the control of eating. Shirley inappropriately tried to control her daughter's eating. Rather than trying to get Jill to assist in controlling herself, Shirley thought she should do it for her. Since Jill was legitimately hungry at times, this action led to Jill's feeling deprived. As a further control tactic, Shirley had tried to cajole Jill into eating new foods for which no taste had been developed. When she wouldn't eat, Jill was forced to stay at the table until she ate something.

Jill revolted after being bombarded with the "good" foods. Jill wanted to eat more of the things her mother would not allow her to have. Fighting continued as each tried to exercise the fullest extent of their power. Each was losing the game but neither gave in.

One major problem in Shirley's plan was that no transition period was used to introduce new foods to Jill. She was not used to some of the foods her mother wanted her to eat. Her mother thought that Jill would become hungry enough to eat them, and they started a waiting game.

Jill was hungry. But rather than eating at dinner, she roamed elsewhere for food. She would find it. Shirley would then become overly concerned with Jill's foraging. Restricting her caused further problems. It was a no-win situation. Although the clamps were down about as tight as they could be applied, food was always available either at friends' homes or at school. Jill continued to gain weight despite extreme restrictions.

Shirley's overconcern with her daughter is somewhat common for parents who have had their own weight problems. This is known as *diet codependency*. Being a devoted parent, she didn't want her child to experience the trials and troubles of overfatness. Unfortunately, the excessive measures were not necessary and caused considerable disturbance in the family. In your own family, you must be careful not to let your expectations taint your approach to weight control. Do not try to excessively control your child's eating or become overly involved in wanting him to lose weight. Go slow, and if you find yourself becoming frustrated, step back and ask yourself, "WHY?"

- Do you have any special concerns about weight control in your own life?
- In what ways could these concerns impact your child or family?
- What are your expectations for this program?

To control weight effectively, we have to know when we are hungry and when we are full. That seems obvious to you and me. But to an infant or young child, learning to respond to hunger and satiety takes experience. Satiety is learned by associating physiological feeling with eating, and then recognizing the need to stop. A key concept in this program is that parents must support children in their effort to learn internal cues that signal feeding behavior. Trusting children to guide themselves in how much to eat, when to eat, and *if* they should eat is quite important for a successful program. Parental trust first evolves from the feeding cycle.

The Feeding Cycle

Feeding is a complex learning ritual for parent and child alike. It is the first time newborns effect in their worlds. As they feed, a negative feeling, hunger, is replaced by a positive result, feeling full. This relationship becomes one of their first cause and effect interactions with the world.

Positive and negative sensations tend to be all that exist in the newborn. Feelings such as happy or sad are not recognized. Since eating feels good, the child repeats eating behavior on a nearly reflexive basis. As conscientiousness arises, actions are paired with situations, which leads to understanding.

With time, infants learn how much to eat, when to eat, how fast to eat. Through trial and error, learning via physical discomfort from eating too much or too little, and the positive reinforcement from food, physical sensations are a form of biofeedback that guide the child's sense of satiety.

Ideally, the child seeks or refuses food on the basis of an internal feeling of hunger. Then he stops eating on the basis of satiety. These internal feelings are physiologically based, not an externally placed demand. Food is used to decrease hunger. Sounds obvious? Yes and no.

Prior to speech, parents learn signs of the various internal cues perceived by the youngster that say "I'm full." Parents must sense when their child needs no more formula.

In the beginning, reading a young child's feeding cues was difficult. Frustration surfaced at both ends of the communication line. An "easy" solution may have been to provide a bottle to "keep him quiet." Giving a bottle became a solution to the specter of a never-ending crying jag. At times, this was not unreasonable thinking. Unfortunately, giving food all too readily can contribute to future problems.

Eating while distressed blurs the boundary between hunger and pain. Regardless of the origin of hurt, food may "help." Time after time, with enough association, food becomes a way to make things OK. So, too, can pain or anger or sadness get confused with hunger.

Physical hunger, the tumbling, nagging feeling of deprivation, often becomes secondary to emotions in many overfat children and teens. Year upon year, the use of food to solve problems escalates. True physiological hunger is misrepresented by emotional reactions. Food for hunger becomes secondary; food takes on psychological meanings.

Most parents recognize that overfatness arises because of poor eating habits, lack of exercise and excesses in eating. But it is more than just that. For many overfat children, food fills spaces it was not intended to fill; spaces outside of the stomach. It is no longer something to maintain life, to make the body work. Food becomes a way to cope.

The Psychology of Food

Hunger is the first of our physiological drives. That's how nature primed us to survive. With such a powerful physical drive for food, considerable pleasure comes from hunger satisfaction. Often, the pleasure surrounding food is used to enhance or assuage all sorts of feelings.

The use of food to enhance happy feelings is sanctioned throughout all cultures. Food accompanies most events, from hot dogs at a ball game to turkey at Thanksgiving. It makes festivities and events more enjoyable, more fun.

Alternatively, when an event is a source of discomfort, some people diminish or distract themselves from feelings through the pleasures of carbohydrates. Food becomes a false solution to problems.

Billy ate heavily on certain days of the week. Thursday night dinner usually ended with two desserts and cookies throughout the night. His parents couldn't quite understand why. Talking with Billy's teacher gave the answer. It seems Billy was eating due to fear of math tests that were always given on Friday mornings. He would become quite anxious about not getting an "A."

Food can be a powerful tranquilizer. Food helps induce a pleasant state of rest. Sugary treats are especially powerful. By inducing delightful feelings of sedation, emotions are given a temporary shove out of the way. Essentially, painful feelings are stashed in the refrigerator or dumped in a cookie jar.

Sue didn't think she was popular enough. In her mind, dieting was the answer. She stopped eating all but supper and exercised every day for about a month. Even after losing four pounds, nobody took notice. She gave up and started to eat more. Within a short time, she put on twenty pounds and felt even worse about herself. But she kept on eating. She said it made her "feel good."

Food is an anti-depressant. People will eat due to sadness, depression or loss. Dissatisfaction with one's self can lead to chronic sadness and excessive eating. Unfortunately, dieting cannot offer solutions to nonself-acceptance.

Louann and her boyfriend had a fight. The first thing she did was to get a large pizza and eat it all by herself. She didn't want to talk with her boyfriend. She wanted to "forget him."

Food hides anger; it's instant comfort in a wrapper. Sometimes it seems easier to run from problems than face them. Confrontation is distasteful. Eating is so much easier when you don't know how to talk about it. Or is it?

Whenever Greg felt tired he would run to the pantry to see what he could find. Tiredness meant he "needed something to eat." He was searching for something to do. Food was an easy outlet. It was "fun" and you could play with it as you ate.

Food is a pick-me-up and a boredom reducer. When "there's nothing to do," all too often food is readily available. Many overfat children would rather grab a snack than grab a game.

When chores were being done, Jane ran for a snack. She didn't like doing housework. Eating helped her to postpone the inevitable. Food helped her to procrastinate. A few minutes of pleasure made daily chores so much easier.

Jim always had to have a bedtime snack. He made his mother get him some treat like cookies and milk. Otherwise, he felt it was "hard to sleep." This routine went on as long as he could remember.

Food becomes a part of our rituals—in these cases, the "put it off 'til later" and the "sleeping pill" syndromes. Food becomes the reason for actions. In the latter, food being paired with falling asleep for so long, the child begins to think food puts him to sleep rather than he puts himself to sleep. Parents must slowly wean children away from these practices.

When Sally would fall or hurt herself, Mom would always give her a piece of candy. Food became a band-aid.

Too often parents will use food to make hurts "go away." Try a hug next time.

When Jimmy and John did well on their report cards, the family went out to dinner and had ice cream afterwards. Soon the two boys demanded ice cream whenever they did good work.

Food is a reward. Since food is a primary need, it is a powerful reinforcer. Due to this fact, it is a natural choice as a gift, reward or motivator. From ancient offerings to the gods for good weather, to today's offerings to a child for a good report card, food has fit the reward bill.

Reward systems should be modified to avoid reliance on food. Attention, money, material goods can be substitutes. Using alternative rewards early in life teaches the child not to self-reinforce with food.

Tammy would often "get under her mother's feet." She would get in the way while her mother prepared dinner. Her mother would call in a baby-sitter—a piece of pie. Tammy would scurry off to a corner of the kitchen to eat. Food kept Tammy busy. A cheap baby-sitter? Tammy weighed over 20 pounds more than her closest classmate.

A little time and attention can give your child so much more. Teach your child to seek gratification without putting a spoon in her mouth.

Tyrone was the "big kid on the block." He lived in a tough neighborhood. He ate to "be big." Size helped to deal with other kids.

Food can help gain power. For example, in urban neighborhoods, where strength is the law of survival, weight translates into a way to cope in places where size rules.

Power also infers attention. One person in my elementary school was bigger than me. He was known as "Big Bill." He seemed to enjoy this notoriety. I doubt it now. He adapted socially by trying to go along with whatever crowd would let him join in. Late in high school he was heavily into drugs.

Often, attention given to the overfat child is negative attention. He may get picked on. It is well known, though, negative attention is better than none. Overfat children may adapt by becoming the "class clown" or everyone's "buddie"—even if he gets taken advantage of. He thinks that then the older children might like him. To maintain his position, he always puts himself down or is quick with a joke, hiding from rejection by trying to be everything to everyone.

Sammy said, "I don't like me." He felt he was a "fatty." His school grades continued to drop as his weight went up. In third grade he was becoming a discipline problem.

Children who do not feel good about themselves may eat as a subconscious banner of low self-esteem. Children who are very shy, who stay away from others, or who talk about being "stupid or dumb" have esteem problems. Overuse of food continues that poor self-image.

As they picture themselves as overfat, eating as an anti-depressant is a way of initially trying to get rid of painful feelings. As weight accumulates, however, the child feels worse. He eats more. Weight adds up—more pain.

It's an unending dance of feeling hurt and getting hurt. Self-esteem further falters as eating intensifies. Eating becomes punishment. His only way out is for you to support him, be with him and LOVE him.

Sasha started to gain weight as she entered puberty. She was an attractive, precocious child. When older boys started bothering her, she turned to food because she didn't know how to handle their advances.

Weight can be used as a defense against involvement in relationships. Relationships can be scary. You risk rejection, hurt or separation. You also receive love, friendship and understanding. But for many older children who are just beginning to explore relationships, the former risks are not worth the latter rewards. It is especially true for those who may have had rejections. To attempt new relationships may provoke fear; nobody wants to be snubbed again.

To unconsciously avoid rejection, weight is a barrier that will stop most approaches from the opposite sex. Overfat children make themselves "unlovable." It's not socially acceptable to like or date the "fat kid."

Overfatness is a "safe" place to be if the budding adolescent doesn't feel lucky in love. Flirtation or other advances from the overfat person are not taken seriously (or at least that is what the overfat person hopes). The overfat teen can "mess around" with the other guy's girlfriends without evoking jealousy. He is not a threat. It comes down to safety in size, hiding behind a wall of flesh.

If alcohol is the adult social lubricant, food is the grease of childhood. The use of food is very often linked with childhood social gatherings, parties, birthdays and holidays.

At your child's next party, see how food is involved. Food is conversation and interaction, much in the same way alcohol serves adults. It gives common ground for interaction.

Both children and adults, however, can get too lubricated. That's when overfatness, among other problems, occurs.

Bobby was one of eight children. He had been gaining weight steadily since sixth grade and was showing signs of high blood pressure. He would eat very heavily and as much as he could. When asked about this he said, "If I don't get it now, someone else will eat it."

Sibling rivalry can lead to fears of "not getting enough." While eating each other's treats happens frequently, not having enough to eat is rare. Reassurance and specific measures to make sure each child gets an equal share is important.

Similarly, although not common, some individuals face starvation every day in this county. When food is unavailable or in short supply, people react physically and psychologically. Seeking behavior becomes prominent. Food is an obsession. Once access to food returns, overeating occurs until weight stabilizes. Unfortunately, in many instances overeating continues.

In cases of extreme deprivation, overfatness presents a psychological "insurance" against future hunger. Future deprivation may never occur again, but the behavior goes on. Extreme examples would be of Depression era individuals and those who went through starvation during World War II. You may have heard of a relative storing large amounts of food for "the next Depression." Some have unconsciously become overfat as a vow never to be hungry again.

Think for a moment.

- **In what psychological ways does your family use food?**

Finally, extreme dieting and specific illnesses contribute to deprivation. Periods of illness, injury or changes in diet may stimulate the dynamics of weight gain. Picky eating, too, can be traced to bouts of illness where foods once relished are now rebuked. It happens because specific foods were associated with being sick. Even if the food didn't cause the illness, a conditioned aversion results. A taste for those foods is lost.

Disruption in eating patterns due to many other causes can fuel the fires of overfatness. Anxiety during moving, changing schools, divorce, family problems or stress lead to more or less eating. As disruption ends, many children continue distorted eating habits. Overeating can become an established pattern.

- **Did anything unusual affect your child's eating habits?**

Many factors cause problems in eating—some are unavoidable, some can be managed. Only with forethought can similar events in the future be approached with minimal stress. So be prepared to make moves or family changes with as much knowledge given to the child as he can handle. Be open and talk.

Chapter Two

First Stuff:
Where Do We Stand?

Your first task will be to observe your family.
•
Style of eating, daily activities and food selections
are what you will observe. Forms are included to
help gather information.
•
Older children can monitor their own behavior.
•
Observations lead to recognizing habits that con-
tribute to overfatness.
•
You target specific habits for change.
•
Subsequent chapters show you ways of changing
those behaviors.
•
Additionally, your child should be examined by a
physician to assure good health.
•
A questionnaire is provided to get further personal-
ized information from your doctor.

"To know what to ask is already to know half."
— Aristotle

Sandra took the observation sheets firmly in hand. She was
not going to allow Anne's weight problem to affect her
school performance. Dan was in agreement. His daughter

was not going to bear the brunt of jokes, jokes so biting as to sour her enthusiasm for school and learning. Sandra and Dan were determined to help in any way possible before overfatness flared into further unforeseen injury. They began by observing her mealtime eating habits.

Sandra selected several days to observe Anne. On Monday, Anne took about 11 minutes for breakfast and around 18 minutes for dinner. Since Anne was in school, no observing occurred at lunch.

While eating at home, Anne would chew quickly, popping food into her mouth, one bite after the other. Food was eaten in large chunks. She did not use a knife or chew very well when eating her meat. As one portion disappeared, she moved to the next. She paused infrequently only to talk about school and TV.

By the way the food disappeared, Sandra suspected that Anne was not particularly enjoying the meal. Anne showed little attention to it as she bulldozed a path across her plate. "How much enjoyment should kids take?" Sandra asked herself. Time was needed to find the answer. Once Anne finished the main course, a large piece of cake vanished along with the last of her milk. While asking to be excused, she slipped off her chair and rushed to her room to play.

Observing on another day, Saturday, Sandra noticed Anne took 6 minutes to mill around her cereal at breakfast. She didn't eat it all before she left the table. Later, 12 minutes were required to drown her tuna fish sandwich in her tomato soup at lunch. The resulting mess was eaten at her mother's insistence. As the last drop of soup drained away, Anne was gone. Sandra heard the TV click on. "Is this how Anne has been eating all along?" she asked herself. Apparently so.

The dinner bell rang in the evening. Anne reluctantly came to her chair. Shifting in her seat, she picked at her meat and vegetables. Very little went into her mouth. She kept asking her mother, "What time is it?" Anne wanted to leave the table 12 minutes after beginning. She was told to stay. She slid back into her chair with a sour frown. Dan asked her what was wrong. She spouted back that she had things to do. "What?" he asked. "Muppets!" she said. Anne was being lured away from the table by the beckoning of her favorite TV show. It was quite evident by this time that TV had some unrecognized magic effects. With these observations, Anne's eating habits were becoming clearer.

Shirley had been frustrated in her own attempts to get Jill to stop eating. She was ready for another approach. She took the sheet on Activities. She glanced at it from top to bottom. It was time to take a look at what was going on here.

Shirley, Dave and Jill fancied themselves an active bunch. Movement was no stranger. The family frequently took long weekends camping in the mountains. They could be seen hiking a trail to their campsite, where upon arrival, they set their tent—a fortress against the moods of Mother Nature or at least a condo in the woods. Time melted away while hiking from hill to peak and back. They were out of doors and felt this was good exercise. It was. Upwards of six hours were spent each day in some sort of activity. Jill spent 10 hours sleeping and, since home was far away, the rest of her time was given to relaxation. No time fell to TV or school work on camping weekends.

Those weekends were a boom time of activity. However, as the family recalled activities from Monday through Thursday, they were coming up empty handed. Shirley and Dave were a bit surprised. The total amount of their exercise throughout the week was far below that received on weekend treks. By all appearances they were packing a whole week's worth of exercise into two days.

Being very active on the weekends was good. Unfortunately, exercise did not carry over to the rest of the week. Likewise, Jill's activity level was minimal. Her total playtime was about 2 hours per weekday, including two half-hour recesses at school. Shirley and Dave asked, "Was that all?" Yes. By using the activities sheet, they calculated the rest of the day was spent in school (6 hours), with 35 minutes to get ready, 30 minutes to eat dinner and about 30 minutes of chores. But what was going on the rest of the day? Oops! The TV was on about 4 hours each night.

The couple had to ponder the deep question, "How did all that tube time sneak in?" Throughout most evenings, Jill sat, legs crossed, face in hands, on the floor peering at the TV. What's more—so did Shirley and Dave. They recognized that the tube had become a bit of a mindless entertainer for them and an ever available baby-sitter for Jill.

The couple had demanding jobs. Perhaps fatigue had spawned their reluctance to exercise much during the week. That was enough to let the TV bug catch hold. Less and less activity had filled the weeks and years since Jill was born. Alternatively, weekends were perpetual motion away from home. Exercise was far easier away from the TV. Camping weekends were well planned and well orchestrated. Weekdays were virtually frozen in disinterest. What to do now? A better balance had to come between the weekends and the weekdays. Was there a way to get rid of this television tapeworm?

Susan and Bill wanted their sons to be as healthy as possible. Heart disease ran in the family and they saw no need to give it a head start if it could be avoided. They understood that the eating patterns set up early would greatly influence the boys' weight in the future. They also knew that their diet was not conducive to weight control. But nothing was ever done about it before. Now was different. The pump was primed at the school nurse's insistence; it was time for a change. The sheet on Food Selection observation was brought out and they began marking in the slots.

For both boys, favorite foods spanned the globe. They liked almost everything, but did ignore some exotic dishes sampled in a restaurant. Octopus didn't go over too well; snails were a real drag, too. Otherwise, little else fell into Least Favorite categories on their sheets, save for spinach and a few vegetables. Children have a worldwide conspiracy against spinach and a loathing for legumes. These guys were no exception. They could smell out a lentil and pass by with upturned noses. Beyond that, few complaints were ever sent to the chef.

Snacks were the next category on the list. They knew snacks inside and out. Their in-between-meal munching consisted of piles of potato chips, popcorn with a generous smearing of butter, and corn chips of every variety—barbeque, cheese, jalapeno, you name it. No holds were barred on snacks. That being the case, the parents had a hard time pinning down how much snacking was going on. The 12- and 16-ounce contents of those bags dwindled away day after day, sometimes hour by hour. They all had a hand in it.

Drinks were next. Milk was a big consumption item. About a gallon a day was drained away. The parents thought the two boys shared the responsibility for drinking the milk. Each quaffed about eight glasses a day. In addition, soda pop accompanied most snacking frenzies. Bags of potato chips were rather dry. The kids would literally suck two to three cans of soda down their gullets each day; some days, even more. And the boys wanted a soda when Dad had a beer. They were right there keeping up with "ol' Pop."

Since difficulties were arising in seeing who ate what, Susan decided to ask the boys to keep their own records of what they ate and drank at home and school. Each drink and snack was to be marked on a sheet. School lunches were written down on another. Drink and snack sheets were pasted on the refrigerator door as a reminder to keep a tally. The boys accepted the responsibility of doing their "nutrition homework."

Jimmy was discovered to be the bigger eater and drinker. Rather than the two boys plundering the pantry goods equally, Jimmy was having about 25 percent more than John. He had approximately four snacks and sodas for every three that John would have. After a week of regular marking, the parents felt this was an accurate representation of what the boys were consuming.

Last to be noted was eating out. Going out to eat was one thing they all liked. It was a convenient way of getting a break from meal routine, and bypassing dishwashing for Mom. The family went out an average of twice per week. Though not unreasonable, it was a little expensive. What did come to be recognized as unreasonable was that fast food was the main staple: burgers, fries and shakes. Quite a few calories came with that food. Further, Susan and Bill agreed the time saved didn't justify the fat in the food coating young arteries. A lot more time would be lost to a heart attack if the boys kept eating like this during their lives.

The family finished their observation sheets. All the questions were answered. The final verdict: Breakfasts and lunches were not excessive; these meals tended to be well-rounded, without too much fat or too much eating. In contrast, evenings were out of control. From after school on, the boys raced back and forth into the kitchen. They waved to each other as they passed on their foraging trips. Eating took up a good portion of the evening hours. Snacking was nearly continuous. What should they do?

As in these case examples, you should, with a watchful eye, pen in hand and forms at the ready, take a close look at your children's habits and behaviors. Observing them in a systematic way is necessary to give an objective view of what may be contributing to overfatness. By fitting together the pieces of the puzzle, a picture forms of the overfatness forces lying in wait to mire your child in a lifelong struggle. You will ferret out the backstairs influences unique to your family; then slowly but surely stamp them out.

In the following pages you will find three observation sheets: EATING STYLE, ACTIVITIES and FOOD SELECTION. Each sheet has topics and questions to stimulate thought as to what behaviors might need to change. Even though some answers may seem obvious to you, don't be too quick to write.

First, take a look at your family. By watching your child in specific situations, you can see what he really does, what he is really like. You may be surprised.

Some habits are easy to measure. For example, it is easy to time how long it takes to eat, to sleep or to watch TV. Other activities are more subjective. You must note if you think he is chewing slowly or quickly; if bites of food are small or large; or if food is chewed thoroughly or poorly. Make a guess as to what is a reasonable standard for your family. If you find this difficult, observing average weight children can give some hints as to what is reasonable. (You may find your children are not so bad off!) The intent is to get an estimate to act as a guide in your program.

In addition, older children can help keep records and assist in answering questions. Everyone can talk about the foods liked, the amount of time at play or recess, or how much was eaten at school. Use magazines to hunt down the types of foods the kids like. Further, writing on a log sheet at school can help the child to remember and to feel responsible for part of the program. A food log is part of the following sheets. Children can be very reliable—let them fill it out. Don't do it all yourself. Let everyone contribute. These types of contributions give a sense of pride if received in a positive and supportive way.

Make copies of the following forms for each family member. The charting will take time. Observe for several days to know how consistent eating and activities are; compare and note different days. With regard to activities, it is especially important to compare weekends and weekdays; two sheets are given for this purpose. As you know, activities vary considerably on the weekends. Other habits may vary, too.

When you are finished, you will begin an analysis of what you found.

Go to it!

Observation Sheet: Eating Style

*Name*_____

Estimate of time spent at:

    Breakfast_____ Lunch_____ Dinner_____

Chews food: Slowly____ Medium____ Quickly____

Chews food: Thoroughly____ Poorly____

Bites of food are: Small____ Medium____ Large____

Pauses while eating: Often____ Sometimes____
                          Rarely____

Puts down knife and fork: Often____ Sometimes____
                          Rarely____

Seems to enjoy food: Yes____ No____

Takes time to enjoy food: Often____ Sometimes____
                          Rarely____

Plays with food: Often____ Sometimes____ Rarely____

Engages in conversation: Often____ Sometimes____
                          Rarely____

Does other things while eating:

    Often____ Sometimes____ Rarely____

What other things?_____

_____

Need to change some eating habits: Yes____ No____

Observation Sheet: Weekday Activities

*Name*_____

Most favorite activities:_____

_____

Least favorite activities:_____

_____

Time playing or exercising per day:_____

Time in school and/or work:_____
(Including homework)

Time sleeping:_____

Time eating meals:_____

Time watching TV:_____

Time doing chores:_____

Time for other entertainment:_____

Time for relaxation:_____

Others: (specify)_____

_____

Is more exercise needed? Yes_____ No_____

Does he or she complain of boredom or lack of things to do?
    Often_____ Sometimes_____ Rarely_____

In what ways could daily activities be increased?_____

_____

Observation Sheet: Weekend Activities

*Name*_____

Most favorite activities:_____

_____

Least favorite activities:_____

_____

Time playing or exercising per day:_____

Time in school and/or work:_____
(Including homework)

Time sleeping:_____

Time eating meals:_____

Time watching TV:_____

Time doing chores:_____

Time for other entertainment:_____

Time for relaxation:_____

Others: (specify)_____

_____

Is more exercise needed? Yes_____ No_____

Does he or she complain of boredom or lack of things to
do on weekends?

        Often_____ Sometimes_____ Rarely_____

In what ways could weekend activities be increased?

_____

_____

What I Did Today

*Name*_____

Day_____

Time I got up:_____

Things I did (write down how much time you took for each):

School_____

Recess_____

Play_____

Walks_____

Bicycling_____

Running_____

TV_____

Radio_____

Eating_____

Homework_____

Chores_____

Sleep_____

Other things I did today:_____

_____

Time I went to bed:_____

Observation Sheet: Food Selection

Name _____

Favorite foods:

    Meats: _____

    Vegetables: _____

    Grains: _____

    Fruit: _____

    Others: _____

Average servings per day
(A serving is two ounces of meat; one cup of raw or one-half cup cooked vegetables or pasta; one slice of bread; one medium apple or orange):

    Meats _____ Vegetables _____ Grains _____ Fruit _____

    Others _____

Least favorite:

    Meats: _____

    Vegetables: _____

    Grains: _____

    Fruit: _____

    Others: _____

Favorite snacks: _____

Average number of snacks per day: _____

Favorite drinks: _____

Average number of drinks per day (one drink equals 12 ounces):

    Soda _____ Juice _____ Water _____ Milk _____

    Others _____

Estimate of meals at fast food restaurants per week: _____

Your guess as to the amount eaten in a day: scale of 1 to 10
1 — Too little; 5 — Just right; 10 — Too much

    Breakfast _____ Lunch _____ Dinner _____ Snacks _____

Comments: _____

_____

What I Ate Today

*Name*_____

Date: _____

Circle day: Monday   Tuesday   Wednesday   Thursday
              Friday   Saturday   Sunday

Write down the foods you ate:

Breakfast_____
_____

Lunch_____
_____

Dinner_____
_____

Snacks_____
_____

Drinks_____
_____

Anything else?_____
_____

Welcome back. Take a round of applause and a good pat on the back. That was some work. You may have learned something new or confirmed something already known. At any rate, this information leads to the next step.

Analysis of the Problem

Where does the family stand? One, two, or three areas may be a problem in your family. By finding which habits need changing, the battle is half over. Finding solutions and strategies is the next step. As with all problem solving, start with the easiest task and work your way up to ensure early successes. First, let's see how others have done it.

Eating Style

Sandra was ready for an analysis of Anne's eating habits. She already knew that Anne was a fast eater. Her average dinner was far less than 20 minutes. She ate large bites of food in rapid succession. As a result, enjoyment was probably minimal. Many children don't take much time to enjoy eating, but this was too little time spent at dinner. Anne was not displaying table habits conducive to weight control.

In addition, her parents found that dinner was becoming a time for Anne to vent her pent-up frustrations. She took mealtime as an opportunity to rattle off about verbal injustices slung by her classmates. She spoke of being teased and her resultant hidden anger. Some meal conversations would even spark bouts of escalating emotion and unruly feelings at the dinner table. Those feelings were quashed in a show of temper by a clenching of teeth and a downing of gruel. In other words, Anne was not a happy camper — she ate to decrease her discomfort. Once discomfort was deadened with dessert, she was off to the TV.

This scenario has three underlying weight control themes:

1. **Slow, conscious eating helps to avoid overfatness.**
2. **Negative meal conversation causes anxiety and over-eating.**
3. **Meals should not be cut short for the sake of TV.**

Sandra recognized that these points could be applied to her daughter. Anne had poor table behavior, especially since she started school. That was when all the teasing started and Anne began to vent her hurt feelings at the table. Even though she was quite young, and table manners are slow to develop, this would be a good time to start teaching Anne to slow her eating style and increase eating enjoyment. In the meantime, the TV stays off at the dinner hour. Sandra had three areas on which to begin formulating her program.

Back to you now. How fast does your child eat?

The slower we eat, the less we eat. Why? Basically, for two reasons. First, research shows it takes about 20 minutes for food in your stomach to start being digested. Until it has begun that journey, you cannot obtain a feeling of complete fullness or satiety. When your blood sugar begins to rise due to digestion, the appetite diminishes. Feelings of satiety come, in part, with changes in our blood sugar.

Second, eating slowly allows the weight of the food to put pressure on the stomach wall, which contributes to eating cessation. If you're not aware of the physical sensation of being full—that heavy, comfortable feeling—you will tend to go on eating. If one eats quickly, feelings of satiety are more easily masked; overeating is more likely to occur. The longer the eating time, the less usually eaten.

Ultimately, the key to weight control is to be in tune with physiological hunger. As stated in the previous chapter, parents and children alike must listen to hunger. When hunger is absent, *do not eat*. Likewise, when a child says he is full, *let him stop*.

Forcing children to eat teaches nothing more than how to overeat. Eating is therefore learned under duress or command rather than because of hunger. That sets a bad precedent. It is more functional to let the child learn what true hunger is. Let physical hunger be the guide as to whether or not eating takes place.

But you may then ask, "Will he eat enough?" The answer is an unequivocal "YES." Parents often fear that children eat too little. Far and away, most eat too much. You have to realize that your child won't starve. I have never heard of a healthy child who starved or became ill because he failed to eat enough at meals when food was available. It just does not happen. Most parents, rather than worrying about not eating enough, should think about limiting foods eaten too often. More about this later. Remember, all in all, eat slowly!

Ideally, meals should take at least 20 minutes from first bite to the last. Now clearly, not every meal needs to take 20 minutes or more. A bowl of cereal would take about ten minutes. That makes sense. Do not spend energy trying to extend small meals. Likewise, snacks should take at least 10 minutes. Take adequate time with your child to sit down and enjoy all snacks. Given reason, any eating should take as long as possible — the longer the better. If your child is not taking 20 minutes or longer for larger meals, is chewing quickly, or otherwise eating too fast, your first target is to slow down eating.

Slowing Down Eating.

The second question: Does your family take time to enjoy food?

Realistically, young children do not take much time to enjoy their food. They have many more things they are interested in. This is a very normal situation. However, by teaching emphasis on the pleasures of taste or meal satisfaction, less is eaten. Focusing on the flavors, textures, colors and aromas can sensitize the diner toward greater enjoyment. Learning to emphasize taste fosters slower eating as they examine each mouthful. The result is greater enjoyment from less food.

The gourmets of the world have the correct idea. If you have eaten a true gourmet meal, portions are small but are extraordinarily flavorful and satisfying. Meals are a bounty of excitement in small packages. Gourmets eat very little; they enjoy very much. The secret is to take a great deal of time to savor food. Examine the food with a keen eye. Note everything you can about it. Satisfaction comes with the taste and sensation of the food — rather than the amount.

You can lead the family toward greater enjoyment of the epicurean delights placed before them. This assumes, of course, some minor culinary talent is available and food is prepared with style, color and variety. Practice will develop that talent.

Improving enjoyment starts with describing what is being eaten. As experience takes hold, one discovers the nuances of enjoyment. Awareness is of main import. Each family member learns to focus on what he is eating. As you notice more, this, in and of itself, will slow eating behavior. Further, by noting color and smell, taste is improved. The sense of taste is a combination of sight, smell *and* your tastebuds. (Remember how food loses its taste when you have a cold? That's because you can't smell it.) For instance, look at the color and texture. Describe its flavor. What does it remind you of? What does it taste like? What spices are used in cooking? Mmmm! Now you're getting the idea.

In no way is it bad to place emphasis on eating. It *is* bad to overeat. Balance in all aspects of life has its rewards. If your family fails to take much enjoyment in food, your target is to teach food enjoyment.

Teaching Food Enjoyment

Lastly, what activities are going on at the table? Do they add to or detract from the enjoyment of the food or the length of the meal?

Anything that contributes to an air of relaxation at the table should be continued. For instance, conversations at the table can be very productive. They can enhance enjoyment and bring the family closer. It is one of the few times during the week that everyone can be together. Eating together is very important. Closeness and support is maintained by eating together. **Eat as many meals together as possible.**

When you are together, part of the focus should be on the food. Try to develop "gourmet flare" by teaching eating enjoyment. How to do this is further explained in Chapter Three. In addition, topics outside of the meal that contribute to feeling relaxed can be added into conversation. Alternately, negative topics, arguments or venting of emotion should be avoided. If not, eating becomes associated with discomfort. As anxiety increases, eating increases.

Problems or negative topics should be saved for another time of the day. Set aside time to work things out after dinner. See that your family does not regularly engage in negative activities at the table. Problem solving should not become a part of mealtime conversation.

As well as removing negative distractions, one must remove the more mundane distractons from meals. For instance, reading at the table is not a good idea. While concentrating on the written word, awareness of food is lost. Almost assuredly, more disappears from the plate. The same happens when you snack in front of the TV. Before you know it, the bag of potato chips is gone. Keep food in mind as well as in mouth. Finish eating before moving on to other matters.

Further specific tactics and recommendations on removing mealtime distractions are discussed in Chapter Three—Head Stuff. It outlines what to do with your family if you have a trouble spot.

Activities

Shirley completed the activity sheet for Jill. She and Dave found, as expected, that Jill was prone to low-level activities such as watching TV, reading and board games. These comprised a majority of her free time. While they did have a swimming pool, its use was restricted to about four months each year. During summertime Jill used it often with her friends. But this wasn't summer; no pool for the rest of the year. So in the evenings, idle thighs crouched in front of the TV. Her mind was active, but her feet were not. Self-motivated evening activities were minimal.

Jill would do just about anything with her parents— that is, when Shirley and Dave instigated the activity. Likewise, her teacher reported that Jill was active in games with other children in all recesses and physical education classes at school. But she was not one to lead. Usually, she had to be invited to participate. Also, her teacher said Jill did not like to compete, such as in running races or games of skill. Those activities caused frustration because she usually lost. Otherwise, she was open to most activities and was a good sport. She was rather cooperative, energetic and skilled for her age.

Shirley knew Jill had about 45 minutes of recess each day. Jill would be very active playing with the other kids.

Running, walking and ball games filled that time. All were good exercises. The school day provided quality activity to contribute to burning calories.

Next, her parents thought of other ways she got exercise. The local children walked to school, about three fourths of a mile each way. This was a good distance for her age and great exercise. Jill would play with friends after school on some weekdays. Combining the time taken to walk to school, the time in recess and playtime after school, Shirley estimated Jill engaged in three hours of exercise per day.

Shirley and Dave thought this amount was reasonable. They quickly became disappointed, however, when playtime and TV time were contrasted. More than three hours were spent watching TV each day. This pointed out that TV was a major menace to activity—something to be contended with. Otherwise, it was a fairly standard day with six hours in school, eight to nine hours sleeping and one hour eating. The rest: chores, relaxation and other entertainment combined for three hours. That added up to an average day for Jill.

The Weekend Activity sheet showed Jill did much more exercise. It also showed something else: When the family was not away camping, the old TV raised its antenna again. Cartoons were a major part of Saturday mornings. Church was a big part of the day on Sunday. Neither provided much activity. But even after those activities, not much else occurred that could qualify as exercise. That translated to a family conspiracy of lazy weekend repose when not out camping.

Nearing the bottom of the evaluation form, they came to the question, "Is more exercise needed?" Without much thought needed, the answer was a resounding, "Yes!"

Go now to your own observation sheets on Activities. What does your child like to do?

Is he prone to active pursuits like biking, running and playing or low-movement activities like board games, jacks or reading? Is he more likely to watch TV or go for a walk? Is he consistent in what he likes to do?

Children who naturally seek activity are much less likely to become overfat. Research suggests that *low levels of activity may be the number one cause of overfatness.* Excess calories are not given time to accumulate in the active child. As he runs, plays dodge ball, baseball or walks the dog, considerable energy is burned. Bodies become efficient, fit and healthier through exercise. Activity is the heart of fitness. Moderate activity can give your child the edge in weight control.

Next question. What does the family do together?

Activities follow a family pattern. If the parents tend to be less active, the child is less active.

By burning just 100 extra calories per day, a person can lose ten pounds in a year. A vigorous twenty-minute walk per day will burn that extra 100 calories. That's very little effort for some very positive rewards. It is one more piece of evidence that weight control can be attainable even with small changes. And it does not even touch on the multitude of other benfits that come from exercise.

Ideally, a balance between low-level and high-level activities must be struck. Much has to be said for low-level activity. Reading is very valuable. Even TV has some shows of redeeming quality. Each has its place and time. But if your child is overfat and tends toward low-level or sedentary fun, high-level activity must be gradually introduced into his life.

The amount of time in specific activities varies considerably between children. Age, medical condition and physical maturity all have bearing on how active they are. Perhaps just as important is how exercise is accepted in the family. If it is a normal, natural part of family life, a child is very likely to remain active all his life. Finding a level of exercise the entire family is comfortable with will go far in supporting continued weight control.

A goal of over three to four hours (total of all activity from walking to recess) per day is reasonable for most families. Some may do more, some less. It is important not to do too much, too quickly, so that your child feels exhausted. Exercise should be moderate, varied and most of all—FUN!

Consider the following:

- High-Level Activities
  active play
  running
  biking
  swimming
  walking/hiking

Any activity that is continuous and raises the heart rate as well as requiring *heavier* than normal breathing, is considered HIGH-LEVEL.

- Low-Level Activities
  watching TV
  sitting
  listening to music
  reading
  coloring
  playing board games

Any activity that is slow or requires little physical exertion is classified as LOW-LEVEL.

The bottom line is: *the more exercise the better,* as long as it is fun and safe. The more the family exercises together, plays together, walks together, the more calories burned. The more calories burned, the better weight is controlled. Combined with proper eating, you can say, "Good-bye overfatness!"

Less than three hours of total daily *high-level* exercise (playing, walking, running) is ususally not enough for the overfat child of age eight and above. Less than two hours is a red flag that needs attention as soon as possible. Less than one hour of activity indicates a serious problem. Does the family need to do more exercise? Most don't do enough.

Our kids are out of shape. Too many people — children, teenagers, adults — are not physically fit. Most children cannot do a single pull-up or run a mile. The Department of Health and Human Services found that half of the children surveyed in grades 5 to 12 did not get enough exercise to reach a basic level of fitness. And in comparison with kids in the 1960s, a much greater percentage of children are now overfat. The time has come to change these facts.

Your family can become physically fit. A little time and a little effort brings big rewards.

It is not necessary to don a pair of running shoes and start pounding the pavement or go down to the health spa to pump iron in order to get into shape. It would be great if you choose to do this, but I use the word exercise in a much less formal way. For our purposes, the time that people are up and around moving fast enough to cause heavy breathing is EXERCISE. The time spent being active, burning large numbers of calories in feats of strength is EXERCISE. So when you estimate the amount of time in exercise, estimate all high-level activity from play clear up to formalized exercise. Think about any time spent moving.

Keeping this definition in mind then, does you computation for total daily exercise meet a three-hour minimum? Don't overinflate the estimate, but any major activity can have exercise value. Any high-level activity done in the day should be calculated into your assessment.

If your estimate is low and you choose to do an exercise program, it is time well invested. You'll see how to start an exercise program in Chapter Four. Other options are available if a formalized program does not suit your needs. Time spent in some sort of activity is essential for weight control. In addition, exercise promotes stress management, can bring the family together and contributes to a quality life style. Without a doubt, healthier families are happier families. Myriad ways exist to increase daily activity with the right amount of family exercise. By changing some daily habits, you can greatly increase the calories your family burns up.

Look again at the Activity sheets. See what happens the rest of your child's day. Time in school ranges from four to eight hours depending on the school grade. (Don't forget to include recess or physical education class as exercise.) That's a big portion of the waking hours. Normal sleep ranges anywhere from four to twelve hours. Other activities round out the day. Chores, meals, relaxation and that old purveyor of the paunch, the TV, fill the remaining hours.

By now you may have sensed my feelings about TV. Nothing has contributed to the overfattening of America more than TV. Kids and adults watch too much. Does your child? If he watches three hours or more of TV per day, another red flag should go up. It's normal for kids to watch TV. But the more time spent in front of a TV, the less likely weight control will be knocking at your door. TV cannot be the mainstay activity for children. If too much TV is being beamed into your living room, limiting the time in front of the set may be a consideration in your program. TV *off hours* are a good idea for most households. For example, no TV from 5 p.m. to 7 p.m. until dinner and homework are completed.

As you have seen, the idea of the Activity Sheet is to show if any one activity is taking too much time out of the day or interfering with more strenuous activity. Knowledge of an average day can be enlightening. Likewise, the same holds true for what your child does on the weekend. How do activities differ? How are they the same? Once these questions are answered, you'll know if your child is getting enough exercise.

You see an average day. You see an average weekend. Is there enough activity? What do teachers say about his level of participation in school activities? If any of the questions in this section lead you to believe more exercise or activities are warranted, the chapter on Body Stuff will give the specifics of how to put more movement in your lives. Your target behavior is to **increase daily activities and exercise.** If your child is older (above age 8), you may wish to consider **starting a formalized family exercise program.**

Food Selection

Susan and Bill filled out the Food Selection sheet for Jimmy and John. They had an inkling that their traditional Midwest meals were a part of the problem that had caused the boys to become overfat. Together they began to dissect their diet.

While the range of foods the boys liked was quite varied, what was actually served at meals was not. Favorite
foods offered by Susan tended to be rather restricted. The
main staple was beef. The family believed that meals weren't
complete without some sort of red meat. It was not unusual
to have beef up to five nights per week and potatoes sat right
alongside more often than not. Potatoes were baked, french
fried, mashed and boiled; even steak fries, home fries, cottage fries and refries (leftovers) came into being.

Other favorites listed on the sheet included vegetables
like peas and beans, which were eaten once in a while. Salad
was marked down as an edible item, but it wasn't on the
table very often either. Susan and Bill recognized that little
variation occurred in the children's diet, which was a direct
reflection of what the two of them ate.

Items listed in the Least Favorite column on the sheet
were minimal. The boys would really eat just about anything. Even though this was true, the couple had to admit
that anything outside the usual was subject to suspicion. But
the boys learned that from Bill. He was not overly enthusiastic about trying new dishes. Chinese or other Oriental en-
trees were approached with caution: "it leaves you hungry."
Mexican food was too hot: "too many peppers." French
cuisine was disappointing: "not enough to feed a bird." So
few regional recipes made their way to the table.

Next, snacking occupied a big part of the family's time.
Potato chips, tortilla chips, cookies and frozen pizza were
stored up in the pantry. Foraging trips by all family members
caused the stocks to dwindle. Each of the boys had upwards
of four snacks per day. The snacks provided considerable
calories for little nutrition—in other words, they were eating
junk food. The parents did not feel the need to restrict snacks,
as they had not restricted beverages either.

Soda had become a staple of the diet. Each family member had at least two to three per day. In addition, the kids
liked whole milk and caused gallons to vanish each week.
Juice was also drunk occasionally on weekends when a big
breakfast was in the makings. Water was a last resort when

all else was gone. Otherwise, milk and soda were the mainstay for the boys.

Finally, restaurant and fast food visits were tallied. The family was skipping out to the local "fat burger" about twice per week. It was an expensive venture in two ways. One, the food they got tended to have high fat and high salt. It took its toll on young and old arteries alike. Two, it was relatively expensive for a family of four. Shakes, fries and burgers were about $16 — no small change for a working couple.

Pulling all the information together, Bill and Susan concluded that the kids were eating "just right" at breakfast and lunch. Dinner and snacks, however, were deadly to weight control. Excessive intake of calories was occurring during these times. Scaling back eating had to occur after school and in the evenings. They knew where to start.

Now it's your turn. What does your family like to eat?

Of the three areas up for discussion — eating habits, activities and food selection — parents have the greatest ability to control access to foods. Therefore, it is most directly open to change. Since the majority of food is consumed at home, by limiting what is in the cupboards and refrigerator, you can help your children select more balanced meals and nutritious snacks and drinks.

Selecting balanced and nutritious meals is not easy. It takes a degree of knowledge, skill and time. Ultimately, by restricting some types of foods while giving unlimited access to others, you can make a very significant impact on overfatness.

No one food is actually "bad" for the body. However, the more a product is refined, the greater the chance of too many calories being dumped in to increase its consumer appeal and too much nutrition being pulled out to increase its shelf life. Many convenience foods have too many calories to justify the nutrition within. That's what is known as being "calorie dense." Some refined foods are all calories and virtually nothing else: few vitamins, minerals or other elements — just sugar, salt or flavorings. The producer inadvertently refined out the nutrition.

If your children are eating minimally refined foods like fresh fruits and vegetables — great! Unlimited access should be granted to these foods. If they skimp on eating fruit and veggies, you may wish to introduce more and more over time while drawing away from refined products. Not *all* refined products, but most of them. Before you buy any processed food, read the label. If you can't pronounce the ingredients, don't buy it. More about labels in Chapter Four.

If you have a majority of refined foods in the favorite category on your Food Selection sheet, a goal to work for is to **introduce more fresh vegetables and fruit into the family diet.**

How much junk food falls into the Favorite foods category? Some is reasonable for variety's sake. I don't want to give the impression that your family must live like a Spartan army training for battle. But often enough, too much junk finds its way into our children. Children grow accustomed to the sugary treats strategically placed throughout the grocery store (especially at the check-out stand). Studies show that children have a natural physiological propensity toward the taste of sugar. That does not mean you have to indulge it whenever they ask for candy. The key words are *moderation* and *substitution*.

What types of foods are found in your Least Favorite category? Why are they there?

Children are influenced by many things in selecting what they eat. Commercials, peer pressure and attention shape eating patterns. Taste can become secondary. Fashion and fad stir the taste buds, even in younger children. Moreover, picky food preference is increasingly common as children grow up. Taste buds change. At times you must accommodate these salivary swings. Other times you must be firm so that junk foods do not become the main pillar of the diet. You must guide early food selections so nutritional balance prevails.

Other factors can have impact on what a child eats. Illness can tweak a taste bud. For example, one time I became very sick after eating some hot dogs. I don't think the hot dogs were at fault because my brothers did not have the same illness. But because I was eating hot dogs at the time, afterwards I found myself unwilling to eat hot dogs. I could not even look at them for months. I developed a conditioned aversion. After watching my family eat the vile little tube steaks, I was eventually able to accustom myself to eating them again.

Aversion to foods is common. Go back to the writing assignment discussed earlier. Did your child ever have a conditioned aversion to any food? How long has it been since it happened? Will the child eat that food now?

All in all, it is hard to judge what drives childhood food tastes. Even in adulthood different peoples' taste buds work in contrary manners. That's the basis for individual tastes. One person's meat is another person's poison. The bottom line of this section is: *Regardless of what they eat and why they eat it, you have great power in influencing your child's eating selections.*

Meals must capitalize on the food preferences that are nutritionally sound—such as fruit and vegetables. Limits have to be set on those preferences that are nutritionally inadequate—such as junk food and excess meat. Weight control comes by fostering a reliance on low calorie foods that are filling and healthy.

Likewise, snacks should be available which are a natural, filling food. Apples can be just as tasty as cookies. Oranges can be just as sweet as cake. As you get away from sugar and salt, tastes change. Soon it takes much less sugar to make something taste sweet. (Tastebuds take about six weeks to adapt to lower levels of salt and sugar.) Some junk food is permissible, but don't train your child to crave salt or sugar.

What types of snacks are being eaten? Too much junk? Begin by having a stock of substitute foods to be used as snacks if you find cake, cookies or potatoe chips as the bulk of the children's snacking. Open the cupboard doors. Any overprocessed junk snacks in there? What can you do without? If snacking is a problem, your goal is to **change snacking selections.**

View ingredients in drinks the same way you look at snacks. Stay away from sugared fruit drinks and sodas. Tend toward lowfat milk. Zero-calorie mineral water mixed with fruit juices is very good; even an occasional soda is fine. But what does your child do? Too much or too little of any one drink?

If too many flavored drinks or sodas are disappearing into your child, your goal is to **exchange types of drinks.**

Eating out is the last family habit being examined by the behavioral microscope. Many restaurants serve outstanding cuisine. Some do not. Eating out can contribute to good nutritional habits. Eating out, however, leaves you vulnerable to the whims of the chef. It's hard to judge exactly what you get on a plate. The more you know the restaurant, the more you can control the service.

What about fast food joints? Those establishments are getting a little better about what falls on the menu. Thankfully, salad is available in most places. Other low calorie selections are being made available as consumers demand it. They are getting better, but are best avoided. That's especially true if the menu offers all-you-can-eat. That's a danger signal for out-of-home dining. Don't walk through the door. The risks of overeating are greater than the benefits of trying to teach the child control. Find another place.

If you're going out more than once a week, ask yourself, "WHY?" Convenience? How much time does it really save? Price? Think about the long-term health costs. Are you or your children really saving much? Don't fall into short-sighted solutions.

Given all that you have now observed, you need to venture an opinion as to how much your children eat. Estimate what you feel each child eats at breakfast, lunch and dinner. Too much? If so, of what? Then answer the same questions for snacking (bottom of Food Selection). You can compare your expectations with the standard serving instructions in Chapter Five.

The information on nutrition in the chapter on Food Stuff will give you the basics. If you determine that a specific food is a problem, steps for greater control may be necessary.

Should the family consume large amounts of snack or junk food, restrictions will have to be worked out. Perhaps certain foods will be banned from the household. Work with the family to find reasonable limits everybody can live with. Be understanding—but firm.

Families are not democratic societies. The parent must maintain *caring* control. As a parent, your job is to train responsible human beings. Ultimately, children must learn responsibility to survive on their own. This is done by giving *AGE-APPROPRIATE RESPONSIBILITY*—a fancy term for something you do already. You let them handle as much as they can at any given age. For instance, an older child has more freedom than the youngster—the older child can walk across the street by himself. By trial and error (with as few mistakes as possible) you determine how much they can do without being overwhelmed. This goes for personal responsibility as well as choosing what to eat. Give them as much responsibility as they can handle.

A further example: Suppose the kids want ice cream every day. You say "no." A compromise to teach responsibility is to let them choose two nights to have ice cream. The kids can choose the nights—you choose how often. You have given both freedom and responsibility in this one action. They learn compromise, as well as learning weight control. You serve up a life-style change everyone can live with.

For more specific instruction, Chapter Five spells out what to do.

What About Psychology?

Review your writing assignment in Chapter One. Always be cautious to avoid pressuring your child. This often occurs because the parent is concerned with his or her own weight. What do you think about your own weight? Try not to let your expectations defeat this program.

Always remember that you are setting out to change habits. Therefore, this is an ongoing *process* rather than an ultimate goal. First, you need to know which behaviors to target. Second, once targeted, the victory comes in change of *habit* not in change of *weight*. If the habit is changed, weight will take care of itself. Weight is too complicated a matter to worry about from the viewpoint of a bathroom scale.

Review the assignment in Chapter One. In what psychological ways might your child use food?

If your child is using food as a psychological defense, talking about fears, concerns or hurts will help. At first he may be reluctant to talk. Returning with shows of support, hugs, kisses or being together will help the child gain confidence. Show him you care. Be there. Talk. Play. Even if it's hard at times to muster the energy, do it. Praise any and all triumphs. Children need that. We all need that. And today, being a kid is not easy. Being an overfat child is even harder.

Supporting the child is the single most important factor for success in this program or any of life's other endeavors. Without proper emotional support, this program is doomed to failure. Support will render your child a much more confident, effective and healthy human being throughout his entire life.

The Last Task of This Chapter

Before starting to plan your program, I would recommend that your child be examined by the family doctor or a pediatrician. This will help to rule out any physical causes for overfatness and help to get some personalized recommendations for your program. Please talk with him or her. A form with questions to ask the doctor is provided on the following page. It will also be useful as a record for future reference.

Date of Exam:_____   Immunizations:

Height:_____   _____

Weight:_____   _____

Blood Pressure:_____/_____   _____

Medications:_____

Medical Problems:_____

Is this child's overfatness due to a
physical cause?_____

Any reason why the child should not exercise?_____

_____

How much exercise is recommended?_____

Any need for calorie restriction? Yes_____ No_____

Does this doctor need to supervise the program?

Yes_____ No_____

Follow-Up Exams:

Date:_____   Date:_____   Date:_____

Height:_____   _____   _____

Weight:_____   _____   _____

Blood Pressure:_____/_____   _____/_____   _____/_____

Medications:_____

Medical Problems:_____

Notes_____

Summary

You have just evaluated three areas of behavior that contribute to overfatness. These were EATING STYLE, ACTIVITIES and FOOD SELECTION. You now know if one, two or all three of these areas are contributing to overfatness in your family. Use the following checklist to summarize your conclusions.

Target Behaviors

Check the following behaviors that need changing in your family.

1. Eating more slowly:＿＿＿
2. Teaching food enjoyment:＿＿＿
3. Removing mealtime distractions:＿＿＿
4. Increasing daily activities:＿＿＿
5. Starting an exercise program:＿＿＿
6. Changing types of table foods eaten:＿＿＿
7. Exchanging types of drinks:＿＿＿
8. Improving snacking selection:＿＿＿

Now you're ready to specifically plan your program!

Chapter Three

Head Stuff:
Clearing Out Old Habits

Basic behavioral principles are outlined.

•

Tactics to slow eating, to increase enjoyment, and to monitor intake are described in this chapter.

•

Self-instruction is a technique to teach eating tactics. You will show the family how to use it.

•

Games are included to make changing habits an enjoyable experience.

•

Slowly introduce habit changes to help decrease the amount of food your family eats, thereby increasing the degree of weight control.

"Let early education be rather a sort of amusement;
. . . not with any compulsion.
This will better enable you
to find the natural bent of the child."

— Plato

Head Stuff outlines tactics for changing eating habits. By changing how to eat, most children eat less and slow weight gain. As intake decreases, however, the same tactics can enhance enjoyment. Feelings of deprivation are avoided. Weight control skills are taught by avoiding restrictive or punitive methods, and making the process as comfortable and natural as possible.

This chapter begins with a quick course in psychological principles. Don't skip ahead. The lecture will be fairly painless. These five principles will ensure you are starting with a bit of basic knowledge which will make tactics more easily understood.

Principle One: Behavior that is rewarded is repeated.

You probably already knew that. Its true meaning is that we do what is enjoyable (rewarding) and avoid what is distressing (punishing). Again, that makes obvious sense. The harder part, however, is defining what is enjoyable and what is distressing to individuals. Definitions are very personal and frequently hidden among layers of experience. What you find hellish may be heavenly to your neighbor.

Food is a strong reward because it is necessary for survival. It falls only behind air and water as a primary need. Anything considered necessary for physical survival is a primary need. Material goods have a different type of importance. These are defined as secondary reinforcers; common items are money, jewelry, and automobiles. We have no inherent biological need for these—we can't eat or drink them—but quickly learn they have value. If a secondary reinforcement has some personal value, we will work just as rigorously for it as we would for a primary need.

Secondary reinforcements add to material comfort and enjoyment. Enjoyment or reward comes to be known through experience. As our experiences are different, our rewards are different. So what does one do to find out what is rewarding to someone else? You watch him and see what pursuits he engages in. Easy enough, you say? Not always.

Many reinforcements are not readily apparent. It can be especially acute when parents try to decipher what continues certain childhood antics. Some kids will provoke their parents by throwing tantrums. You say one thing, they want to do another. It happens at times with all children. For instance, various and sundry fireworks flare at the local mall; suddenly the whole store full of shoppers have their eyes on you! What makes this type of behavior rewarding to your child? Is sprawling out in front of 40,000 shoppers, feet and hands beating the floor, shrill screeches flying, all that enjoyable? Not likely. The act itself has little payoff. But in most cases, *attention* from the parent is the reward.

Principle Two: Attention is one of the most powerful reinforcers

In the example, the child's histrionics are really a need for attention and control. The need for attention is a formidable desire that is present in all relationships, especially in adult-child interactions. Furthermore, it is so inviting that *negative attention is better than no attention at all.* Unfortunately, misbehavior is a way of getting attention from an adult, and the child's attempt to get his own way. When a child is flailing about, it is difficult to ignore for even the most patient among us. Attention from the adult "feels" good even though the situation is bad.

Logically then, if the child feels the only way to get attention is to cause a fight, the child will often be fighting. Thus, if you wish to avoid fights, don't spend time telling him how bad he is when he has just caused a disturbance. When he's off playing nicely, tell him how good he is.

Principle Three: Positive reinforcement is more powerful in changing behavior than punishment.

Rewards shape behavior. Punishment and negative reinforcement are less potent for change. Punishment, as you know, occurs when an action is followed by a negative event. A bad grade on a paper means no TV for the night. That's punishment. Alternatively, negative reinforcement occurs when an unpleasant event is turned off by some sort of action. A parent keeps yelling until the garbage is taken out. The garbage goes out, the yelling stops—that's negative reinforcement. The two are very different ways of shaping behavior through unpleasant means.

Since rewards are more powerful than either punishment or negative reinforcement, and they avoid emotional fallout, a reward approach should be used. And it must be as consistent as possible.

Principle Four: Inconsistent or delayed consequences cause change to develop more slowly.

Consequences should be regular and immediate. If you want a child to eat slower, you praise him as he is actually doing it, right at the table, right away. As the child sees the association between your praise and eating slower, he is more likely to eat slower now, and the next time. The more reinforcement, the faster the change and the stronger the habit.

Finally, to get the changes started, you and your spouse should model the behavior.

Principle Five: Children imitate the behavior of adult role models.

Kids mimic adults. Children follow many of the behaviors found in their parents. For true change, any transformation you wish to see in them should be displayed in your own life. If you want them to slow down, you slow down. Do they need more exercise? You do more exercise. Show, tell and do it yourself. Praise them as they follow along. Eventually, through time and practice, better habits will form and weight control becomes a greater part of daily living.

Behavioral Tactics

Modeling will be used to teach weight control. You will show your child how to learn by example and help to shape the habit by praise and attention. As time passes, reinforce and maintain the new habit by periodic observance. Within two to six months (depending on age), adoption of the new habit occurs and the child displays more self-control.

Goal One: Slowing Down Eating

The basic tenet of eating control is to have a reasonable portion of food, enjoy it to the maximum possible and stop eating when full. That's all common sense. The act of heavily focusing on food is not so you have more, it is so you have *less*. The object is to eat and enjoy, but the message always in the back of the mind should be to eat reasonably. Overindulgence leads to a loss of pleasure in the meal. Anything that detracts from a meal is avoided.

Here are some hints to set your family on the path to slower eating and greater enjoyment:

- Keep meal and snack times as consistent as possible. Try to eat at the same time each night. Likewise, plan snacks for approximately the same time, morning and afternoon.
- Meals should exceed 20 minutes and snacks should exceed 10 minutes.
- Take a deep breath and let it out slowly before you start eating. Meals should not be rushed. A deep breath will allow you to begin to relax.
- Review what is to be eaten at the meal before everyone starts to serve himself. Know exactly what you are eating.
- Take small bites. Chew thoroughly. Note all the flavors and how the food feels in the mouth. What does it remind you of?
- Put down utensils occasionally. Enjoy each morsel.
- Eat until halfway finished then take a break for a minute. Ask yourself how you feel. Are you getting full?
- Continue until reasonably full. Let the body signal you when you have had enough. Eating is to get rid of hunger. Is the family really eating because of hunger? Or for some other reason?
- Leave *something* on the plate. Do not leave a sparkling clean plate. Save the food or throw it away. Get away from the old myth that you are doing a favor for starving persons in some remote village by eating everything. Eating too much only hurts you. It doesn't save a soul.
- Make a reward chart or calendar that will be used to display rewards given for game performance. Reward tokens can and should be awarded to the children participating in the following section of the program.
- Set rewards for game performance. Immediate verbal praise is given all the time. Also, tokens awarded can be redeemed for items like movie passes, toys or outings in the park. Tell the children how many tokens are necessary to receive a reward.
- When addressing the child, be sure to have his attention. Speak directly while looking into his eyes. Explain exactly what you would like him to do and why. For instance,

"Billy, I don't want you to have that candy because it is not good for your health." Be very matter-of-fact and firm when necessary.

Teaching Through Modeling: Self-instruction

Younger Children: The Good Eating Game

Self-instruction is a technique developed by psychologist Donald Meichenbaum to help children contend with many types of problems, from academic difficulty to lack of impulse control. By reviewing his extensive research, I have attempted to adapt his treatment model to fit weight control. It has very positive applicability to overfat children. Through my own experience, however, I have found it helpful to use a game as a fun way to teach self-instruction for slower eating for children under eight years of age. Kids have short attention spans; you have to make learning enjoyable.

I have not found it terribly important that the younger child know that this game is an attempt to slow his eating as a means for weight control. He may misunderstand or misinterpret your meaning. Many times when well intentioned parents attempt to explain in detail, the child becomes confused and feels he is doing something wrong. This is a game for the family to play for fun and health. Let natural curiosity take its own course.

When ready to start, tell the entire family you would like to play a new game at dinner time called the Good Eating Game (or whatever you would like to call it). Make sure your spouse understands what's going on before you start. It will be just like "Simon says," only you will say "Mother says" ("Father says" for those industrious Dads out there) and everyone does what she does. But if you don't say "Mother says," then they should "freeze" and not do anything.

Say, "Now follow along and those who do well will get a star each night. Three stars win a prize. But remember, do what I *say* and not necessarily what I *do*. Any questions?" When you sit down to eat, each family member will follow your lead.

Everyone has sat down with his plate at the table.

For example, you say, "Mother says take a spoonful of corn." Everyone puts a spoonful of corn in his mouth. Next, "Mother says chew slowly." They chew slowly.

Continue on, alternating with different foods. Make sure they are eating slowly and tell them how they're doing.

Then, for instance, say, "Take some meat." If someone takes meat, stop him. "Oops! I didn't say Mother says!"

To add further variety, the parent should say one thing and do another. Let the children catch you in what you're doing wrong. Say, "Chew slowly," but chew very fast. An extra point goes to the person who caught you. And so on. Keep going back and forth. Make it challenging.

Work through half of the food on your plate. As the family understands the game, shift to Dad or an older child. "Mother says Dad take over." Dad proceeds to play just like you did. If time permits, each child in turn can be the leader.

Remember to praise the child if instructions are followed. In the beginning stages, it is very important to give feedback to the children. Make sure they know that slow eating is important. After a few successful rounds say, "Mother says the game ends for today." Afterwards, congratulate each other for a job well done and give a star for the chart. Unless a child refuses to play, each should get a star for following at least half of all commands during every meal played.

Run through the game at a number of meals on different days for a few weeks until it is clearly understood. You may choose to stop for a few days. Invoke the game at any time you see family members eating quickly. Let each person lead during a meal to further reinforce learning.

Periodically, fall back on the game to help foster good eating habits. Use it whenever necessary and adapt the game to suit your family. You may wish to do it differently than I have presented. Feel free to change it. The variations are unlimited; find one that best serves your family and entertains your children. Slowly but surely, eating slows in response to your prompting and the practice provided by the game.

Self-instruction for Older Children

Pre-teens and older children can profit from self-instruction training. Sitting down with the older child, it must be made clear that the *entire* family is going to engage in tactics for weight control. Self-instruction will be one part of control that works by slowing eating, which diminishes weight gain. Let him understand that it is a way of getting more from his food, a method of enjoyment. Since this is always a serious topic, parents should approach the child with support and kindness so he does not feel singled out or alone in this quest.

The basic self-instruction steps are:

1. Take a deep breath and slowly let it out.
2. Survey all the food on your plate. Note what it is, the color, the amount. Know exactly what you are eating.
3. Take note of the aroma of each.
4. Take a *small* fork full of *one* item. Place it in your mouth.
5. Chew it thoroughly. Note all the flavors and how it feels in the mouth. Take a moment, then repeat.
6. Put down utensils after every two bites. Chew and enjoy each mouthful.
7. When half finished, take a break for a minute. Ask yourself how you feel. Are you getting full? Does it taste good? What do you like most?
8. Continue eating until reasonably full—not stuffed— then *STOP!*

The above steps break down the eating process into explicit steps. It's the same as if you were driving a car with a standard transmission for the first time: push in the clutch, put transmission in gear, let out clutch while giving gas, and so on. Soon, driving becomes easier and smoother with practice. The same process of learning is going on here.

Go through the steps with your famiy. Talk through the basic format. Understand and memorize it. While doing so, ask if anyone has any suggestions as to changing steps or doing it differently. If a good suggestion is proposed, change the sequence. Make the steps as personalized to your family as possible.

In the beginning of self-instruction, provide positive feedback to the child for slower eating. You can run through the steps during a number of meals. Together, recall and apply the steps. During as many meals as possible—breakfast, lunch and dinner—the parents should take turns in reviewing the steps for a minimum of five minutes. All steps should be said aloud and everyone follows the instruction. As the children retain the sequence of steps, let each have their turn at leading, too. All the while, parents should give positive verbal reinforcement for good performance and monitor each child's slower eating. Don't punish the child for not doing well. Only tell the child when he is doing *well*. Say nothing negative regarding his eating habits.

Once you are convinced the child knows the steps, move the overt instruction to more covert understanding. This is the tricky part. The object is to keep the child eating slowly by getting him to silently say the steps to himself. The spoken steps evolve to become internal commands as the child monitors his own eating. In order to do this, the parent must assist in continuing to provide periodic positive feedback as the child eats slowly.

The child may adopt self-commands such as, "I watch how fast and how much I eat" and "I want to eat slowly." This is the development of internal self-talk for eating control. He says the steps silently to himself just as if he was talking to someone else. Where you first had spoken the steps aloud to everyone, the child now verbalizes the steps silently to himself. You may test his self-talk by asking, "What are you thinking?" This cues the child to recall the self-instruction steps. Use this same question when you see the child's eating speeding up. When he responds with an appropriate answer and slows down, praise him.

Ultimately, you hope to guide the child to reinforce himself, as well as being rewarded by you. As you tell him he does well, he tells himself the same. Tell the child to congratulate himself. As experience takes hold, try to get him to reinforce himself more and more. Since self-reinforcement is slow to develop, you must be careful not to allow your children to fall back into old habits. If they slide back, increase your own verbal rewards until awareness of eating returns. As you might imagine, this is a very difficult task for some children to complete. Don't get discouraged. You are changing a tremendous number of behaviors, so it will take time and continued cueing to remember self-instruction.

Another factor to consider is that the resultant behavior might not be exactly correct. For instance, chewing has slowed but big bites are still being eaten. That's OK. Tell the child what he is doing correctly. "That's very good for slowing down." Tell him specifically what behavior is correct. As time goes along, you can shape further change.

After slow eating becomes habit, encourage him to take smaller bites. In a supportive way, ask the child to recall as many rules as possible. Ask him if there is anything missing. If he recognizes that he is taking large bites, congratulate him. If not, ask, "How big should our bites be?" If he answers correctly, give appropriate verbal praise and reinforcements.

When the above suggestions have been put to practice with good consistency, you can move toward traditional table activities without beginning with continual self-instruction review. You may seek to change other aspects of mealtime behavior. Take conversation, for instance. Mealtime conversation can be conducive to weight control with some simple preparation and preplanning.

Structured Conversation

Structured conversation modifies table talk to foster good eating habits, as well as being a sharing time for information and events. You probably already do it in part. Mainly, conversations at meals should be light, interesting and free of anxiety or conflict.

Keeping table talk stress free helps keep eating under control. The focus remains on the meal and is not diverted by volatile emotions. As emotion and anxiety increase, eating becomes associated with discomfort. That leads to overeating. Meals should be hot, tempers should not.

Problems should not be worked out at the meal table. Call a family meeting later in the evening to work out any differences. Tables should not be miniature battlegrounds. If battling continues, separate the warring parties using TIME OUT as explained in Chapter Seven. Strike a truce until later.

Make dinner a forum for closeness in the family. It's one of the few times the entire family is together, so try to eat together as often as possible. Use the time to talk about how your children are doing in school or in other activities. Listen to what all family members have to say. Understand what they think. Know what is happening in their lives. Communication can greatly improve harmony and success in this program—as well as in other ways.

One way to keep conversation light and free of conflict is by having prearranged topics for discussion. For example, start your meal in this way.

1. Pray, if you are religiously inclined.
2. Preview what will be in the meal. Take a few minutes to explain what is on the menu.
3. Take a minute to review the self-instruction tactics for slow eating. (This is optional, unless it is early in your program.)
4. Start the family conversation.

Topics should include:

- Standard information: what happened at school, at work or at play.
- Something new learned that day.
- Positive events of the world.
- Guessing games—different foods, drinks, dishes of the world.
- An assignment: For example, the night before, the family agreed that they wanted to know something. One person is assigned to find out about it.

    Assignment Ideas: A new book. Why is the sky blue? Names of animals in the zoo. All about the moon. How do planes fly? Countries of the world. What are the food groups and what foods come from them? Etc. Periodic review sessions. Go back and repeat program exercises as needed.
- Any others you can think of.

In summary, the concept behind these tactics is to make eating habits explicit and mealtimes as enjoyable as possible. In order to control weight, a person must be aware of what he eats, how he eats, and know when he is full. One must acknowledge feelings of fullness and use them to stop eating with as little interference as possible. Thus, unconscious habits become conscious control.

As you teach awareness, the children begin to recognize their internal limits. Stopping becomes more spontaneous. As they progress, feelings of competency and effectiveness arise. Self-instruction becomes second nature and good habits take a firm foothold. With time, the habits become stronger and feel natural. It is simple but effective. The hard part comes down to the three magic words: practice, practice, practice.

Other Stuff

A few other habits contribute to weight control. As you may recognize by now, no one single habit change is going to bring total control. Many little habit changes contribute to the overall picture. Some of these are:

Visual awareness

As eating awareness is the goal, it's important to avoid activities that block visual awareness. Children need to see to understand size and volume. Without the eyes paying attention, children (and adults) have a hard time estimating how much has been eaten. Activities that block vision substantially interfere with awareness.

For instance, no reading at the table. By concentrating on the stories, one can easily lose sight of how much is being eaten. Kids fall into the trap of being lulled into overeaters' storybookland. What they gain in literary competency, they lose in weight control. Also, enjoyment is lost if the focus is away from the meal. The eyes never alert the mind to measure the culinary cargo about to be shipped in. That's not what weight control is about. The best policy is no reading, writing, drawing or TV at the table during meals.

Environment

Surroundings are very important. Meals should be in familiar places. Being in the same area night after night helps one to remember the rules of eating and to eat less. Sights, sounds or smells help us to recall. Avoid eating in multiple places if possible. Having a designated eating spot where all meals occur would be ideal. It narrows the opportunities for extra munching.

Getting rid of eating in the bedroom or in front of the TV would be great, too. Many a chip has vanished during reruns of "The Three Stooges." Think about how many occasions you started with a full bag of your favorite munchies and ended with a wrapper. That's not encouraging. You and the bag just got junked.

We have grown accustomed to eating all over the house. Once, a long, long time ago, people had places called dining rooms. All eating occurred in these rooms. Today, however, dining rooms are more show pieces than functional places — modern day museums and art galleries. Rarely do we use them for dining.

Even if you don't have a dining room, you may wish to begin to restrict the places where food or snacking is allowed in your house. Granted, it is nice to have a snack in front of the TV. As long as it is not an everyday practice, it won't hurt. But if you find your kids eating in front of the TV each night, you have something to think about. You may want to restrict the number of nights snacks can be eaten in front of the TV. Maybe they would agree to stopping all together. Possible? Try it! At any rate, eat in as few places as possible.

Special utensils

You may want to have special utensils for the children. Get plates that are smaller than normal. Food looks bigger. It seems like you are eating more than you are. Try it yourself. Food seems to have more volume. It works especially well with children.

Get a special setting for each child and let him be responsible for caring for it. That helps him feel this is an important undertaking. It also helps you with doing the dishes (a nice side effect). Special settings will help cue your child to remember his tactics. And buying a new setting could be a reward for doing well in the program. The significance of that place setting really helps the child keep all his new habits in mind. Some parents have even taught their children to use chopsticks during oriental meals. They slow down eating and can be a challenging task of manual dexterity.

Plate preparation

Responsibility for obtaining food on the plate can be given to older children. In preparing to sit down to a meal, the older child can take that new place setting and learn to serve himself. *All foods should be kept off the table.* No family-style service. Take the child over to the food on the counter and let him put together what he wants. Furthermore, you can show the child how to fix his plate using the same self-instruction process learned earlier. By talking himself through the serving process, he takes command. You can model it for him. Try this:

1. Look at all the food. Ask yourself, "What do I want?"
2. Take an amount, then put some *back.* If you want more—seconds are available.
3. Ask, "Have I taken a little of everything I need? Is it balanced with all the food groups?"
4. If so, take the plate to the table; if not, balance the plate with the correct servings.
5. Sit down and dig in—using slow eating self-instruction.

It's that easy. The child can fix his own plate. One thing implied in this is that children should be allowed to obtain the amount of food they want. *They should pick what and how much to eat.* This notion may seem counterproductive to weight control. That is not true. The best way to get a child to control his weight is to let him determine what and how much to eat. By what you have placed on the counter, you make sure he selects from vegetables, fruit, dairy products and meat. Selections have to be made from what you put out. Ultimately, he can't go too far wrong. This will be further discussed in Chapter Five.

Guilt

If you use guilt to control eating in yourself or your kids, it's time to stop. Guilt has been associated with weight control more than any other emotion. No longer. Guilt is a very negative way of controlling another person. It is very similar to punishment. You do something wrong and you feel bad. As you know, punishment is a much less effective way of changing habits.

Stop the "guilties." If you find yourself or your mate attempting to use guilt, look at control from another angle. Understand that every decision made has some costs and some benefits. We all can make *any* choice affecting our lives—eat more or eat less, exercise or play cards, do homework or watch TV. Some choices are better in the long run while others are more immediately satisfying. Children tend to choose immediate satisfaction because it's hard to wait. The here and now is more important than the future. But they develop the ability to delay gratification with time. One eventually learns he cannot have everything at any given time.

With the child's increasing maturity, you can influence the development of delayed gratification. By pointing out the costs and benefits of choices, children can develop a greater sense of eating control and personal responsibility. By outlining consequences (positive and negative), the child learns to associate actions with outcomes. Those outcomes have a reward and a price. For example:

Do I want cake?
What are the costs and benefits?
      Costs = weight gain, low nutrition, dental cavities
      Benefits = taste good, "fun," sugar high
Which is more important, costs or benefits?
Make a decision without guilt.
Pay costs—receive benefits.

Guilt is taken out of the equations because costs and benefits are recognized and paid. Let me illustrate further. I eat cake on occasion. I do not feel guilty. If I want it, I will have it. I never fully restrict myself from *any* food for *any* reason. (You set yourself up for failure in seeking the forbidden fruit.) But I do not have cake very often, as the costs are too high. So if I eat it, I enjoy it. I take time to savor it.

Then I have to pay some costs. I may run a little farther that day to burn off the extra calories I just ate because

I do not want to gain weight—some benefits, some costs. If there is no time to run, I choose not to eat cake. I judge whether its worth the costs because I have made a commitment to myself for weight control. Again, I have cake if I want it. But in remembering my commitment, I do extra exercise to pay the price.

Of course, younger children do not think in these terms. Only after abstract thinking arises does full understanding occur. But pre-teens can understand specific examples with your guidance. The cost and benefit equation breaks down if costs aren't paid. As I set costs for myself, you can set costs for the child. The tough part is not turning it into punishment.

Paying costs through exercise is the best method for weight control. If the family had a large meal, that was the choice, and that was OK. No guilt. But now you must pay some consequences if you ate more than you needed and don't want to gain weight. The best family decision is to go for a walk (after waiting 20 minutes for digestion). Let the walk be a positive and enjoyable experience so it does not take on the flavor of punishment. Stroll off to your favorite park to burn those extra calories.

Talk to your older children about the costs and benefits of eating. If the child chooses something, talk to him about the choice. If cake is chosen, ask him why and what the costs and benefits are. Regardless of what is said, congratulate him on his thinking ability. Then plant the idea that, at other times, he may not choose cake because of the extra calories and other costs that he must pay to keep his weight under control. Together, go off for a fun walk. Likewise, go for a walk at times even when he does not choose the cake. Reward him with some time together. Avoid giving the impression that the walk is punishment.

Even though children will often choose cake for immediate gratification, the eventual association of the costs will improve their decision-making. Time will provide a path to understanding choice.

In addition, to help decision-making around high cost items, you may limit access on certain days. For instance, don't completely ban dessert—have it only two nights per week. Let the kids choose which nights. If dessert is requested two nights in a row, that's it. No more for that week. Better planning might come about in the future if they find themselves for want of dessert later in the week. That is delaying gratification; that is learning costs. What other reasonable costs can you think of?

Can you think of any other habits you would like to change in the family? Do any other changes need to be made with respect to eating habits? Take a few minutes to review your notes.

Back to Anne, Dan and Sandra

Sandra read through the chapter titled Head Stuff. She told Dan about self-instruction and how it is used to slow eating and increase enjoyment. It seemed workable. The two of them decided it was time to start.

The family sat down before dinner. Sandra told Anne she had a new game to play. Everyone could win at this game and would receive stars for good performance. The stars were to go on a calendar. After getting three stars, that person could choose a special dish or surprise at the next meal. Special rewards were won once anyone received six stars.

Sandra showed Dan and Anne how the game was to be played at dinner. The two agreed to play. They chose to call their game Slow Byte. The name came from the new-found love of computers Dan and Anne shared. Byte was computer jargon. Sandra made the rules and steps of Slow Byte.

The game was played at dinner time when everyone would be present. Sandra memorized the basic self-instructions. She started the meal by relaxing. She encouraged Anne and Dan to follow as she said the instructions aloud. She went through each step: chewing slowly, being relaxed, focusing on her food. She mentioned every step in one form or another. She challenged Anne and Dan to listen carefully.

Before the first meal was over, Anne was picking up instructions. Sandra would quickly praise and reinforce her. Anne learned some of the steps and wanted to take over. "Take small bites, put down spoon." Dan got caught. "I didn't say 'Anne says.'" The first meal went well. Anne and Dan received stars.

The next night began with a review. Sandra started off and Anne and Dan followed. Having gone through only once, Anne took over. She stated how to take slow bites, chew it up well and try to feel full. She picked up on most of the steps. She showed immediate signs of being more aware of eating.

This initial game was played during most dinners for about two weeks. They would change it around, such as guessing which step one of them was doing. When Dan was gone on a business trip, Anne still would recite the steps to her mother to get stars. Anne was able to memorize all the steps and apply them consistently in a short time.

To add greater variety, each family member would take turns starting off and rewarding stars. Also, Sandra prepared some new recipes to practice slow eating on new foods. Most foods tasted good, and Anne, Dan and Sandra got their stars as new dishes were tried. Anne and Sandra even walked to the library to get cookbooks for new recipes. Enjoyment went up as eating went down.

As habits changed, greater rewards were given. Anne was quickly filling her calendar. They all put their heads together to think of a reward. Anne eventually got some athletic shoes she wanted. As she continued to do well at meals in the upcoming months, Dan decided she would win that new bicycle she wanted. They could ride bikes together.

After it became apparent that Anne knew the steps, they periodically added structured conversation. One of the main topics surrounded working on the computer. It was the hot topic in the home. Everyone wanted to learn to use the computer, so "computer talk" was spoken at the table. Once in a while, conversation turned to eating habits to assure compliance on everyone's part. In addition, Sandra and Dan wanted to make sure Anne was reinforcing herself for eating slowly. If she remembered the steps, she got more stars. The game was invoked when Anne's eating got faster. After two more months on the calendar were filled, she got the grand prize. Dan picked out a computer program for her.

About eight months later, they looked back to assess how they had done. It appeared everyone had slowed down on eating. It was clear that less was being eaten and the enjoyment from what they did eat was increased. Occasionally the game was called up. Eating was slowed down again and the habits were getting stronger. In addition, walking had become a stable part of the nights when a big meal filled the table. Costs were paid when necessary to burn off those extra calories. For the most part, emphasis was placed on the quality of food rather than the quantity, and the family devoted themselves to much more exercise than in the past.

Sandra found that Anne slowed her rate of weight gain. Since her height was catching up, she was looking better. She felt better. Anne further reported that the children at school were not picking on her nearly as much. School problems were ceasing. That was the most welcomed news to the parents.

Mom and Dad lost about 10 pounds each, too. They felt good about that. All in all, their program was deemed a continuing success. The commitment to change was made. There was no sliding back from here.

Chapter Four

Body Stuff: Play Ball!

Half of all children get too little exercise.

•

Many benefits come from exercise. Exercise *must* accompany any weight control program.

•

Under age six to eight, formal exercise programs are not necessary. Play activities can provide ample exercise.

•

Older children can and should have some sort of exercise program that is fun, challenging and varied.

•

Fitness entails proper body composition, flexibility, cardiovascular endurance and strength.

•

When exercising, one should warm up slowly, exercise for at least 30 minutes and then take time to cool down.

•

Exercise should occur at least three times per week, every other day.

•

Have realistic goals. Chart the progress of your child. Reward hard work.

•

Most of all, have fun!

———

*The notion of "no pain, no gain," should
be equated with "no brain."
Exercise should be fun, varied and without injury.*
— Archer's Law

A recent study suggests that half of all children fail to get adequate exercise. Why? For many reasons. In part, because of the advent of modern conveniences and little heavy work. Our technological world has reduced labor to a minimum. We have shifted from being an agricultural society to being service oriented. Machines do the work people once did. That's fine for progress and production—it's not fine for burning calories and staying in good physical condition.

Children have access to entertainment that requires little or no effort on their part. Take television. TV has been a blessing and a curse. It has brought a world of information to the average person that was unimagined before its introduction. It has opened so many avenues of information and entertainment that it has also spawned convenient excuses to avoid exercise and activity. Long periods of inactivity fill the day as the tube burns late into the evening hours.

This is TV's inherent flaw. It doesn't require any energy. Save for getting up and changing channels, no muscles are used. And remote controls have now done away with that bother. Since children and teens tend to spend so much time in front of the tube, and they're doing it more every year, activities and exercise have been in a continuous decline since the first TV was brought into American homes. We even find the main activity for some children is television; up to six hours per day. That is far and away too much. Occasional TV is acceptable; too much assures inadequate exercise.

Families must take responsibility for increasing activity. And they must take responsibility quickly because further studies suggest that since the 1960s, the bodyfat content even in average weight children has been rising. Kids are carrying more fat, and we know more are overfat than just a few years ago. This trend must be stemmed for the sake of our children's health.

Poor exercise habits learned in childhood are carried over into adulthood. Unfortunately, that can mean that even if your children are not overfat now, it still could easily happen later in life. In adulthood, not knowing how to control weight eventually leads to "middle-age drift." Our metabolism slows with each decade after the 20s due to loss of muscle tissue. If eating and exercise changes don't adjust for the decreased need for maintenance calories, overfatness may have an opportunity to rear its head. The best way to avoid it is to become comfortable with exercise in childhood.

Exercise has myriad benefits. It reduces stress, lowers blood pressure, increases high density lipoproteins (removes cholesterol from arteries), decreases depression and makes you feel good. You say that's great for adults, but do kids need protection from stress, high blood pressure and cholesterol? Yes!

Studies on Korean and Vietnam war casualties showed men as young as 19 had some signs of arteriosclerosis (mild hardening of the arteries). It sounds hard to believe. That's too young! But it's true. It points out that heart disease prevention must start early—the earlier the better. Now pediatricians are much more careful in monitoring blood pressure in children. They start at age three; you should too.

Exercise is an absolute must in weight control. Dieting can lead to loss of muscle tissue, strength and tone. Dieting alone cannot work for long for this reason. Exercise prevents the loss of muscle and speeds use of fat tissue in metabolic processes. If exercise is not done, weight control is like the burden of Sisyphus. Once you push your rock to the crest of the hill, it will eventually roll back down on you. Help your child to burn more calories and retain strength through exercise; dieting alone will not work.

We are finally getting research evidence that proves exercise can extend life. We knew it enhanced quality of life; now we have evidence that it can do more. What this boils down to is that it is never too early to begin to get the benefits of exercise and activity. Choosing an activity and staying with it is the challenging part. So what can your family do?

Activities

Most exercise for young children (under age eight depending on physical maturity) should come in the form of unstructured play. Doing what they want, any way they want is the kind of exercise best suited to this age group. Kids need to play. They need time to be kids. So when I refer to exercise for young children, playtime *is* exercise. They don't have to be out pounding laps around the track. That may come later in life. But for now, don't make them grow up too fast.

Under age eight, structured activities should be de-emphasized. A regular exercise routine is not necessary. Play will provide the necessary running, jumping, moving. Playtime: encourage it, praise it, engage in it with them. Play as much as possible. Encourage activities that take a great deal of energy—that make them breathe hard or move quickly. Play is nature's way of conditioning children.

Beyond play, you can do other normal activities that contribute to fitness. Do anything that uses up more calories. Since modern conveniences contribute to overfatness, you can remove some for better health. Use your creativity. Here are a number of ways of increasing daily calorie usage. Try any of the following:

- Use the car as little as possible. Walk with your child to the store, school or park.
- When you have to use the car, park it far away. Walk farther to the store by parking across the lot.
- Plan family walks in the morning or evening. Take the dog along.
- Use stairs whenever possible. Don't take the elevator.
- Go to the park. Go somewhere where the kids *avoid* TV and can play together.
- Find active games you and your children can play, for instance, hide and seek, tag, kick the can, softball catch.
- Take a bike ride.

- Make housework more interesting. Make a game of it. If the child is willing to help, he can get an extra half-hour of your time to play anything he wants.
- Go hiking or backpacking together. Take a vacation that involves a great deal of exercise. Go to a health resort.
- Get a hobby you all can share that will use up energy. For example: collecting leaves, rocks, fossils.
- Others you can think of.

For those interested parents, infant and young children's exercise classes are available. Again, these should not be the main focus but can add greater variety to fun activities. Dance, aerobics and gymnastics are typical offerings. Contact your local YMCA/YWCA or university to see if such programs are available in your area. Parents must be careful in what to select and in what to expect from these programs. Some parents believe structured programs can give children special advantages. They can. Programs contribute to children becoming comfortable with exercise. If not pressured, and slowly introduced to different activities, children are more likely to exercise in the future. Essentially, they become more accepting of activity and exercise.

You cannot, however, accelerate motor coordination and development. A child has to mature to do that; it's physically, not motivationally based. Difficult games or activities that are beyond current abilities can be frustrating and cause the child to turn away from exercise. Maturation comes only so fast. Get enjoyment out of exercise. Don't try to outdo the kid next door.

Activities for young ones should provide a great deal of freedom to have fun. The teacher should ask the class to follow along but not rigidly expect each child to exactly conform. For example, a teacher says "jump" and the child can use his left or right leg to jump. "Wave arms" and the child can do it any way he wants. Fun! Simply said, classes must be supportive and run by a knowledgeable professional. Make sure you evaluate the coach's skill in relating to the children, and his effectiveness as a teacher. Those teachers graduating from the American Coaching Effectiveness Program (ACEP) have taken a course that can greatly enhance their coaching abilities. Has your coach taken such a program? Look carefully at his or her credentials so that your child has a good experience with sports.

Swimming can be a sport to start early. Occasionally, parents begin before the child is out of the cradle. Some think the child will be "drown proofed" by starting so early. No child can be drown proofed. You can make the child comfortable with water—but don't ever trust young children alone. Children under three years of age that start swimming should be closely supervised. Some points to consider are:

1. Their heads should not go underwater.
2. Water temperature is warm enough to avoid chills. Avoid very hot water as found in jacuzzis or hot tubs.
3. Measures are taken to control fecal contamination.
4. Instructors are qualified and know CPR.
5. Infants with medical problems should have physician approval.

When these measures are taken, the child can learn the joys and thrills of water play. Swimming is still not completely possible for young children; but play is. The swimming skills will build with age. And as with all forms of exercise: Enjoy!

Exercise and the Fitness Foursome

Older children (over age eight) can engage in limited exercise according to age and maturity. Formal exercise will not harm the healthy child. Exercise needs to become a more acceptable part of childhood. It can be, as long as it continues to be fun, well managed and injuries are avoided. Only then will exercise be a lifelong pal; only then will the child receive long-term benefits.

Exercise and fitness go hand in hand. Exercise moves the child toward fitness. But what is fitness? It's a combination of four things: *body composition, flexibility, cardiovascular endurance* and *strength*. Body composition has been discussed since the introduction. Fitness implies a relatively low percentage of bodyfat; below 25 percent or so for elementary children. Low bodyfat further implies that a good portion of muscle is on a child's frame. That means being relatively lean, but being strong. Lower bodyfat denotes better health when not taken to extremes.

The second aspect of fitness is flexibility. Flexibility is the ability to stretch or make muscles lengthen. The more flexible, the better the fitness. Flexibility varies greatly. Some people are naturally more flexible, although no one is "double jointed." These rubbery people are just more flexible. Additionally, good leg and back flexibility can help to avoid injury or low back pain. By taking time to slowly stretch *without bouncing,* most people can greatly improve flexibility.

Cardiovascular endurance is the third facet of fitness. This is the body's ability to deliver blood and oxygen to muscles for work. The more efficient or better shape you are in, the more oxygen is delivered. The more oxygen, the more work your muscles can do and the greater tolerance toward exertion is available. Your body performs longer without fatigue.

Endurance includes the delivery of oxygen to the heart, one of the most important factors in being able to exercise (or live). People who do lots of exercise that requires heavy breathing (aerobic exercise) improve cardiovascular endurance most effectively. Failure to increase the heart rate during exercise is not effective in increasing overall cardiovascular endurance. Your heart must pump a little harder and your lungs must breathe a little faster to become fit.

Finally, strength completes the fitness picture. Strength is the ability of muscles to contract. The more contraction in a muscle, the more it can move. Large, muscular people have more muscle fibers. The more fibers, the more strength. Exercise causes muscle fibers to grow. It also makes them more efficient so that strength increases quickly in a person beginning a program. Work toward moderate increases in strength. We're not setting out to make a new generation of Mr. and Mrs. Americas.

The moral of fitness is: BALANCE. All people need a balance of stretching, cardiovascular and strength exercises to be in the best health possible. If you do not use your muscles, you lose 'em! Your body will revolt without proper exercise. Don't cause a revolution—EXERCISE!

The Road to Fitness

Before your family chooses an exercise program, ask yourselves the following questions:

- What do we want or like to do?
- If it's new, can we learn it?
- Can we afford it?
- Do we have the time?

These questions will help you to select a routine. But before settling on an exercise program, make maximum use of it by:

Goal setting. Write down specific goals. Have realistic goals that the family can achieve. For instance, walk a little farther each week. Expect to take anywhere from six weeks to six months to get into shape. Take your time and don't do too much too quickly. The fastest way to turn everybody off to exercise is to do more than each can handle.

Plot progress. Make a chart of what the children do each week. Display it. Put the chart in a place where everyone can see how much he is improving and how much farther it is until the next goal is reached.

Exercise together. Staying together helps hold motivation and interest. Everybody gets into shape together.

Reward improvements. Acknowledge to the family when exercise is "working out" and everyone is following through on attaining reasonable goals. When the goals are reached, give out some prizes like sports equipment or new athletic shoes. Continue to set new goals that will contribute to further success with exercise.

Try a variety of activities. Try anything once, even if the family is not sure they will like it. You may be surprised to find fun new games. You might not be able to start your own polo team, but seek and try new activities.

Put a list of activities on the refrigerator. When the children reach for a snack, it will remind them (and you) to do something else.

Since balance and variety are the keys to success, I'm going to present a number of exercises for possible inclusion in a routine. Maybe you can think of more. Regardless of what you choose, make it fun, challenging and safe.

Starting Off With Flexibility— Stretch 'em Out

All exercise activities must begin with a warm-up. Warming up prepares the muscles for exercise so that injury is avoided. Injuries occur because of neglect. There is no excuse for a child or an adult getting injured. Take your time. Know what you are doing and teach it well.

All exercise begins with stretching. All stretching should be done slowly with *no* bouncing. As you begin to stretch, take a deep breath and let it out slowly. Do each exercise, working from head to toe. Stop immediately if any pain is felt at any time.

1. *Head circles.* Roll the head to the left for 5 complete rotations. Now the other direction. Loosen the neck.

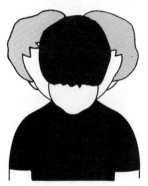

2. *Arm circles.* Hold arms straight out to the sides. Make big circles in each direction, 5 to 10 times. Flex those arms.

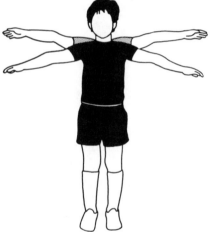

3. *Waist circles*. Hands on waist. Bend forward, to the side, backwards, and then to the other side, 10 times in each direction. Stretch those sides.

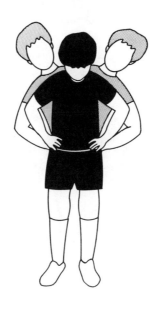

4. *Toe touches.* Slowly lean forward with knees slightly *bent.* Stretch downward as far as possible. Hold for a 3 count. Then back up. Do 5 times. Stretch the legs and back. Be careful not to jerk or bounce.

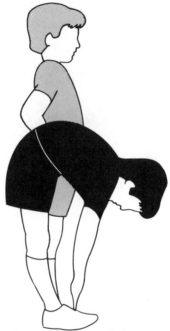

5. *Leg stretch.* Sit on floor with legs spread in front of you. Stretch out with fingers to touch toes on the right foot. Hold for a 3 count. Same with the left foot. Repeat 5 times with each leg. Feel those legs stretch? Great!

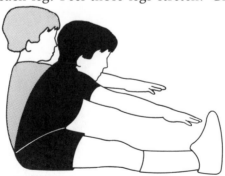

6. *Survey your body.* Any tight muscles? If so, stretch them out. Take your time. Hang loose, shake out the tension. Stretching will improve your flexibility fitness.

7. Use other stretching exercises you like to do.

Take a slow run for about 30 to 50 yards. Raise your heart rate. Now you are properly warmed up.

Cardiovascular Training or Keep 'em Breathing

All exercise should occur a minimum of three times per week for 30 minutes, preferably every other day. This insures adequate conditioning and time for muscles to recover to avoid injuries. It is possible to exercise moderately five days per week without ill effects in the healthy child. Of course, fitness comes faster with more effort. Really vigorous exercise, however, should not occur more than four times per week. Chances of injury increase proportionately as intensity rises. The harder you work, the greater the possibility of injury and being turned "off" to exercise. So take it easy!

Before children work out, they should always have adequate rest (8 to 12 hours per day) and good nutrition (see Food Stuff) to aid in recovery. A further precaution for vigorous exercisers: Children do not get rid of heat as well as adults. If the family is going to be doing extensive exercise or it's *hot* and/or *humid* outside, make sure the kids have plenty of water. Let them drink as much as they want before, during *and* after the event. No salt pills either, please. They are not necessary for athletes at any age. We get more than enough in our diet.

Exercises

Walking. One of the best exercises for anyone is walking. Children can walk long distances with little chance of excess fatigue or injury. Walking speed can be easily adapted to the child's ability. As he walks briskly, heart rates increase to fitness producing level.

Five miles is not an unreasonable distance for healthy, older children to walk as a long-term goal. The entire family can engage in walks in the evening for any comfortable distance. A typical schedule would be to meet on Monday, Wednesday and Saturday and walk a predetermined course.

Find a course that is reasonable for your family. Try it out and see if all members can walk it without major difficulty. Don't forget to pay attention to safety. Walk the route and time yourselves. Once a time is determined, try to beat it. Set an interim goal. Don't start out after five miles immediately. How fast can the family go? Plot progress on a chart. Reward yourselves once your goal is obtained. The faster you improve your time, the faster fitness benefits accrue.

Walking, like other exercises on hard surfaces, should be done with proper shoes. Get a good pair of walking or running shoes. The shoes should have deep padding and an arch support. Skimping on shoes only leads to sore feet and knees. What price do you put on pain? Talk to your shoe store owner about moderately priced walking shoes and buy them. More about shoes later.

Roving. Roving is the marriage of walking and running. It is especially suited for children who do not have the endurance to sustain continuous running. The child may determine ahead of time how far to run, then walk, and then continue running. For example, run a distance of a quarter mile, then walk a quarter, then run. Alternate back and forth. Likewise, you can do the same with time limits. Run five minutes, then walk five minutes. Keep alternating. When starting off, it is best to run until moderately fatigued then walk until breathing recovers. Start running when breathing is back to normal. Combine running and walking to get the benefits of both.

Running. Running is truly a joy for those who start slowly through the "break-in" period. Many families start too fast, too long or too much. They get turned off and quit before any benefits arise. Learn to love running, but build the relationship slowly.

Running, as does all exercise, produces profound effects. Running is my personal choice for cardiovascular training. Your family, too, can discover its brand of wellness. Much of America has come to respect it, as the running "fad" has outrun its fad status. Running is here to stay.

Children between the ages of eight and 12 can run from one to three miles, three times per week. Your child must experiment with distance to find what he can do comfortably. In order to motivate toward longer distances, more children are looking to racing to provide the push. Training for races is a good way to keep running motivation high.

Two-mile Fun Runs are offered more and more by running organizations to fit the distance needs of the pre-adolescent. Any child under age 12 can compete with proper training. Running races are very popular today. Two-mile Fun Runs are a distance that children can tolerate. They must run consistently for two to three months, three times per week, to get into shape before racing.

Distance Training: The Specifics

If this is your family's first introduction to running, start with a distance of one half-mile or less, three times per week. Run it slowly, building up speed until it is easy to do. After three to six weeks, extend the distance. For instance, make the course three-quarters to one mile. Keep running. After another three to six weeks, increase to one and one-half miles, and so on. When the children are running uniform times for two miles, go to your local running shoe store for details on the races in your area. Send in your application for the Two-Mile Fun Run and have a good time!

For children over age 12, longer running events are becoming more and more accepted. A very popular race is the 10k or 10,000 meter race (6.2 miles). It's not an unreasonable distance. By training correctly, many pre-teens, adolescents and adults are capable of running a 10k. Again, training is the key.

Training must be systematic and realistic. By slowly extending the distance run, you can work up to the 6.2 miles necessary to finish the race. As before, go a little farther every few weeks. If the child is just beginning to train, expect that it may take six months to get into shape so as to finish the race. Remember, *finishing* is the object in early racing. Don't get caught up in trying to beat anything other than your own previous times. Have fun!

As your child continues to train, if his intent is to win, work toward increasing training distance to eight miles. Run eight miles at least once a week for ten weeks. This is so the 10 kilometers feels easy to run. Then go for speed. Try to improve times and keep running. The children may eventually win awards for their age groups at the race. Medals are usually given for several children's age groups. Good luck!

Marathons. I rarely run races longer than the 10k. It is not necessary to go beyond that distance for most adults. Unless a child is exceptionally mature and able-bodied, he should not race beyond the 6.2-mile mark, either. Marathons are for special adults. As you can guess, the training involved is extensive and challenging for a person expecting to run 26 miles.

Furthermore, some research suggests that very heavy training can hurt the ends of the long bones in children's legs. As the bones are still growing, they tend to be soft so they can expand. That's how we grow taller. The constant impact of very long distance running can hurt those parts of the bones. It can cause pain and, perhaps, longer-term problems. Some medical researchers feel marathon training could hurt growth. We just don't know for sure. Shorter distances are OK, but avoid the marathon.

A Note on Equipment

Shoes. Shoes are the most important equipment for a runner. Running causes from three to five times the body-weight to impact on the bones. Shoes help to absorb that impact if heavily padded. Many companies make excellent shoes to take that force. You have to find the shoes that will best suit your family and your budget. Good shoes will ensure a long and happy running relationship. Bad shoes will leave a painful mark on a running program. Fit shoes carefully. Help your child find the best pair.

The heel should not move up or down in a properly fitting pair of shoes. Blisters will erupt if the heel rubs. Pull the strings tight. If the eyelets are close together, the shoe is too big. Find another pair. There should be one quarter to one half inch of room in front of the longest toe to the inside tip of the shoe. Your child should be able to wiggle his toes. Have him try on both shoes. Do they rub anywhere on the foot? If they don't feel good now, they never will. Try another pair. Running shoes don't "break in" much.

Find a pair that are comfortable in the store. Let the aspiring runner take a spin on them in the parking lot to make sure. Get a good pair. Yes, they cost a little more. It may be what you consider expensive. But it is worth it. And reserve the shoes for running. Don't let those expensive engineering wonders get torn up by daily use at play or at school.

Clothing. When running or performing aerobic exercise, your family should dress in layers. As they warm up, the layers can be shed.

How much to wear can be a problem. You've got to balance being cool at the start, while not being too heavily dressed as heat builds from exercise. Running really heats up the body. The rule of thumb for clothing is to wear what would be comfortable if it were 20 degrees warmer. For example, if it is 60 degrees outside, wear running clothes that would be comfortable if walking around outside in 80 degree weather. Running is hard work. The heat must escape. Don't overdress, and drink plenty of water. You'll all feel better.

Bicycling. A very good alternative to running is bicycling. The impact of running is absent in biking. It's a good way to see the countryside, too. More distance is covered, so some find it less boring than running. Since you are using muscles you don't use in running, the combination of running and biking keeps the legs in top shape. Most of the leg muscles are given a great workout when doing a little of both exercises.

In determining a distance to ride the bike, four miles of biking equals one mile of running. Biking is more efficient, so you must do more to get the same effect as running. As always, observe safety rules and ride *with* traffic. Obey the same rules as if you were in a car. Make sure the family knows those laws.

Swimming. Swimming is one of the best overall exercises. It works the entire body. It is second only to cross-country skiing in producing fitness. Furthermore, you stay cool and have no impact on joints. It's a near perfect exercise, but you need a high level of skill to continuously swim. You also need a pool, which costs a few dollars. But overall, it's great. If your children have access to a pool, please get them to use it. If they don't now how to swim, see about lessons. Even just playing and splashing in the pool is great fun and good exercise.

Use the pool to stimulate exercise. For instance, see if you can challenge each other to beat his or her *own* record for laps. Challenge on the basis of beating your own record—not each others. Everybody wins, everybody enjoys.

For comparison purposes, one mile of swimming is equal to four miles of running. In turn, one mile of swimming is equal to 16 miles of bicycling. Exercise distance equivalents increase by a factor of four. Swimming is four times harder than running and 16 times (4×4) harder than bicycling. Swimming is potent exercise. It is hard work to move through the resistance of the water. That resistance makes it a top exercise.

Strength — Muscle Mania

Strength training rounds out the fitness four. Strength exercises help to build individual muscle groups, whereas cardiovascular training enhances generalized fitness. Strength requires short bursts of concentrated force. Cardiovascular endurance requires continuous lower level energy output. Both are necessary depending on the demands placed on the body. Here are a few things your family can do to improve strength:

1. *Push-ups.* Lay face down on the floor. Place hands palm down at shoulder level. Push up away from floor until arms are extended. Lower your body to the floor for one repetition. Keep going. If the child can't do it on his toes, have him do it from bent knees. Keeping knees on the floor, push up and return. Start with 10 to 20 per day. Do more if possible.

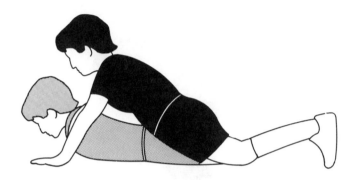

2. *Sit-ups.* Lay on back. Bend knees with feet flat on floor. Cross your arms over your chest. Sit up as far as you can while exhaling. Lay back slowly while inhaling. Do 10 to 20.

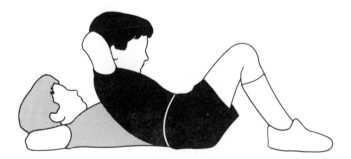

3. *Bar pull-ups.* Mom and Dad hold a bar over the child that won't break under his weight. Have the child hang as long as possible. If he can pull up toward bar, then do so. Otherwise, hold on as long as possible. Do one to 10.

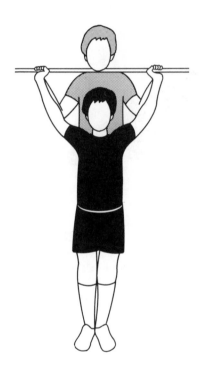

4. *Arm curls*. Get a book or heavy object. Hold it next to your side. Curl the object up toward the chest. Let it down slowly. Repeat 10 times for each arm. As it gets easier, use a heavier object.

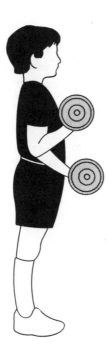

5. *Bench Press*. Lay on back. Hold heavy object over chest. While exhaling, push object out till arms are fully extended. Return object to chest and repeat. Do 5 to 10.

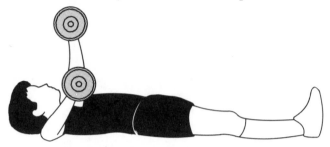

6. *Overhead press*. Stand tall. Hold one book in each hand, hands at shoulder height. Press arms straight out overhead, exhaling. Return and inhale. Again, press overhead. Do 10 to 15 times.

7. Can you think of any others?

Cool Down

After all that work, the family needs to take a few minutes to cool off. Don't immediately sit down. Walk around swinging your arms and shaking out any tightness. Cool down gives time to relax muscles and let the heart rate go down. This is also a good time to do a little more stretching. Sit down and stretch out. Don't just plop down somewhere without giving yourselves some time to slow down from the exercise. Now give yourselves a big pat on the back. Have a drink of water. You've all done well!

When Hurts Happen

Pain and injuries should be guarded against. This is best done by planning for safety, warming up properly and not overdoing the exercise. Some aches and pains normally occur. But if a severe pain should occur, go immediately to your doctor and *follow* the advice given. Of course, it is always best to try to avoid injury by not going overboard. The old saying "no pain, no gain" is wrong. The right one is "no pain, still gets big gains." If any of your family feels pain, STOP! Don't push it. Allow yourselves to rest. If it continues, take a few days off. After resting, start up slowly. Work the family back with continuous, moderate exercise. Take time to get back into shape.

RICE is the answer to pain. Not the grain, but Rest, Ice, Compression, Elevation. If you get hurt—rest. If there is swelling, place ice on it and rub out the pain. Afterwards, elevate the injury so the fluids can drain back into the circulatory system. Most of all, REST and see your doctor if pain persists.

Activity for Shirley, Dave and Jill

Lack of exercise was a major reason for Jill's rapid weight gain. She spent too much time in sedentary pursuits. Shirley saw this at the onset of her evaluating Jill's activities. More activity was certainly necessary. How could she increase exercise and help Jill slow her weight gain?

Shirley recognized that Jill would work for attention. Furthermore, Jill would do most of what Shirley wanted as long as it did not concern eating. Shirley immediately began to walk to the store with Jill, even if only a single item was needed. Shirley attempted to walk with Jill whenever they went to the mall, to grocery shop or to school functions.

While this increased Jill's caloric output, her mother was feeling enthusiastic about starting an exercise program. Walking became a daily occurrence. Monday, Wednesday and Friday became family walk days. All three members of the family set out on a mile-and-a-half course.

The parents paced themselves so that Jill led the walk and she could stop momentarily if she became tired. Walking continued for about five weeks. As they got into shape, walking became faster. Later, a two-mile course was set and they started to work up speed again. The miles were melting away along with some extra calories.

Shirley kept a record of the distance traveled. For the most part, lap times continued to get faster. They started with 18 minutes per mile. When they reached the 15-minute mark, Jill received new walking shoes as a reward. Walking continued as long as the warm weather held out.

When fall and winter set in, strength exercises were tried. Each family member did the warm-up and strength workout. They added a few exercises and walked at shopping malls on the weekends. After a while, they were greatly increasing the push-up and sit-up totals. They were becoming stronger month by month.

As motivation was bustling, they decided to go to the university to lift weights and ride the stationary bicycles. Three times a week they met. It was a nice change, and seeing others working out helped to keep up their own routines. The parents met with a fitness instructor to learn about weight lifting. Jill took swimming lessons in the heated pool. Swimming was something that felt good. She could hardly wait for summer to get into her own pool with her friends.

At one point, Dave had to leave for a business trip. After returning, the family was lax in continuing with the workout program. With a little prompting, they eventually got back on track to their previous fitness levels. By varying their routine, interest remained high until summer arrived.

Shirley felt Jill's weight was getting under control. Ten months later, Jill was looking much more fit, felt better and had lost two pounds. The weight loss was very significant as she had grown nearly two inches in height and had lost a few inches around her waist. In the past, she would have gained much more during that amount of time. The exercise program was having definite impact on her weight control. Everyone decided "working out" was here to stay.

Summary

Fitness is comprised of body composition, flexibility, cardiovascular endurance and strength. In order to become fit, one should slowly warm up with flexibility exercises. Follow with 30 minutes or more of walking, running or other cardiovascular exercise and throw in some strength exercises for good measure. Finish off with a cool down. Vary the routine as needed. Keep up the work. This amounts to a job well done and a body well kept. Exercise, exercise, exercise!

Review your notes and summarize your plans for exercise in this final sheet. Go on to enjoy the world of exercise —for a lifetime!

• What are some tactics to increase daily output short of formal exercise?_____

_____

• Does your child need a formal exercise program?

Yes_____ No_____

• Favorite activities: Walking_____ Running_____

Swimming_____ Biking_____ Other_____

• Exercise Schedule

	Mon	Tues	Wed	Thur	Fri	Sat	Sun
Activity:	____	____	____	____	____	____	____
Time:	____	____	____	____	____	____	____
Goal Distance:	____	____	____	____	____	____	____

Chart daily distances to see how you all are doing.

Walking Chart
(Example)
Month: June
Distances

	½ mile	1 mile	1½ mile	2 miles	2½ miles	3 miles
Dates: 1						
2						
3						
4						
5						
6						
7						
8						
9						
10						
11						
12						
13						
14						
15						
16						
17						
18						
19						
20						
21						
22						
23						
24						
25						
26						
27						
28						
29						
30						
31						

Chapter Five

Food Stuff: What's for Dinner?

Nutrition is the process by which the body uses food.

•

The basic building blocks of food are proteins, carbohydrates, fats, vitamins and minerals.

•

The six food groups are milk, meat, fruit, vegetable, grain and junk.

•

Children should have three servings of milk, two of meat, at least two of fruit and vegetables and four from the grains each day.

•

Buy foods that are fresh or close to the natural state; fewer nutrients are lost and fewer chemicals are added.

•

Read labels carefully to know what you are buying.

•

Style of preparation greatly affects the final caloric content of a dish. Avoid frying. Use baking, broiling, boiling, and microwaving.

•

Snacks are an important part of nutrition for children. Have two or three snacks a day. However, avoid junk food whenever possible.

•

Go to a restaurant where you really know what is in the dish. Avoid fast food.

•

Bon Appétit!

> *"Beware of those foods that tempt*
> *you to eat when you are not hungry*
> *and those liquors that tempt you to*
> *drink when you are not thirsty."*
>
> — Socrates

Nutrition is the process by which the body uses food. Food powers all the body does from thinking to moving. Food provides the building blocks for each and every cell. Food is the basis of life. It is vitally important, but as with all aspects of life, too much of a good thing is a problem.

Nutrition is not difficult to understand. It is a matter of checks and balances. Once the basic terms of nutritional balance are known, excess calories are avoided and weight stays within a reasonable range. (Weight always fluctuates day to day; weight can only be thought of as a range rather than a single number.) With practice, children can select a balanced diet to assist in weight control. A balanced diet will help ensure weight remains reasonable.

Major Nutrients

Food selection is the art of presenting the body with adequate nutrition for optimum health and weight. We all need certain nutrients to be healthy, to grow and to prosper physically and mentally. Food is comprised of five major nutrients. These are **proteins, carbohydrates, fats, vitamins** and **minerals.** Each has its own role in the body.

Except for water, **PROTEINS** are the most abundant compounds in the body. Protein is the brick and mortar of all cells. Cells, in turn, are the building blocks of all people. Proteins are necessary to replace and increase the number of cells and are the "glue" that repairs damage.

Proteins are built from amino acids. Twenty-two amino acids combine to make specific proteins. Eight of these acids are considered "essential" because, unlike the other 14, these eight cannot be manufactured by the body. Since the body cannot make them, they must be supplied by the diet.

Animals are made from the same types of cells as people. All amino acids are contained in their flesh. When meat is eaten, all amino acids are obtained for use by the body. On the other hand, plant amino acid structure differs from animal proteins. Since plants are not as complex as animals, most do not contain all the essential amino acids. Therefore, if you are a strict vegetarian, you must carefully combine certain vegetables and grains to get all the amino acids in correct balance. Beyond this, no hard research supports the idea that combining certain foods helps you to lose weight or "cleans" out your body.

CARBOHYDRATES are the sugars and fibers that come from plants. Carbohydrates are the main source of energy in the body. Forms of these sugars range from simple to complex, depending on structure and chemical detail.

High fiber cereals are slowly digested. In fact, most fibers can't be completely digested by humans. Our digestive tracts are not able to break down very complex, water-soluble fibers like grass or bran. But fiber is very important. It adds bulk to the diet. Bulk facilitates absorption of excess bile (cholesterol) and aids in waste elimination. It helps to keep us regular.

Digestion takes longer with complex carbohydrates. Before carbohydrates can pass through the intestinal wall, digestion must break them into smaller sugars. Since it takes time to break carbohydrates down, sugar absorption through the intestine is slowed. The resulting blood sugar rise is slow. That's good because moderate levels of sugar slowly infusing into the vessels retard feelings of hunger. This is what's known as having a high satiety value. In contrast, if you have ever eaten a candy bar and found yourself hungry ten minutes later, you will understand what I'm talking about. Candy has low satiety value.

Carbohydrates such as candy cause a rapid blood sugar increase. Candy does not require much digestion. It quickly passes through the stomach wall, and its sugar is dumped into the blood stream. Rapid blood sugar increases cause a release of insulin. Insulin pours into the vessels and starts doing its job. It vacuums up excess sugar, placing it in storage. Unfortunately, the insulin may be so efficient that blood sugar may drop too low. You then feel more tired than before eating the candy. You are now experiencing the "sugar blues." Eventually the low blood sugar trips a physiological alarm; a sudden lust for carbohydrates returns.

Because candy has a low satiety value, you need to eat again soon or your blood sugar will remain low. That candy "pick-me-up" has just put you down. Many calories were taken in—and no feeling of fullness results. Thus, rapid rises in blood sugar are to be avoided. That is best accomplished by eating fruits, vegetables and grains in a natural state without added sugar. Staying away from processed carbohydrates will help everyone feel less hungry when learning to control weight.

The next component of food is fat. **FAT** is a vital part of body cells and structure. Some fat in the diet is necessary. It performs many functions in nutrition such as supplying fatty acids for cellular activities and transporting specific vitamins. We can't live without it, but we can live with less.

Although fat is necessary, we generally have far too much in our diet. The source of excess fat is usually meat or whole milk products. Eating less red meat and whole milk, thereby reducing fat intake, is a worthwhile goal for most of us.

VITAMINS AND MINERALS perform as partners in the building and repair of tissue. Small quantities of these substances also provide the push behind metabolic processes, without which we could not survive. Vitamins are not magical substances. They help do what the body does normally. Large doses don't cure anything—other than the drugstore's financial problems. Very high, continuous doses can be harmful or fatal to children.

Vitamin A is necessary for the growth of all cells, especially those lining the body. It keeps us healthy and resistant to infection. It also aids in the adaptation to low-light vision. Vitamin A comes from liver, carrots and green vegetables.

Vitamin B1, also known as Thiamin, is necessary to utilize carbohydrates. Without enough B1, the energy process is thwarted and you cannot use food properly. Thiamin comes from cereals and meat products.

Vitamin B2, or Riboflavin, is also needed to metabolize carbohydrates and fats. It's found in milk products.

Vitamin C or Ascorbic Acid, has been widely written about. Basically, this vitamin helps hold cells together. Your cells can almost fall apart without it. It plays a vital role in keeping tissue strong and resistant to infection. It does not, however, cure the common cold, at any dosage. You get Vitamin C from citrus fruit and green leafy vegetables.

Niacin is like the other two B vitamins. It aids in energy production and comes from meat and grain products.

Calcium is a mineral. It combines with proteins to build the skeleton. Bones and teeth need plenty of calcium to be strong. Other nerve processes need it, too. Ninety-nine percent of the calcium in the body is in the bones. Everyone needs calcium throughout life, especially women and girls. Lack of it leads to osteoporosis, otherwise known as brittle bones. Calcium comes from milk products and green leafy vegetables.

Iron combines in the blood to carry oxygen. The oxygen is released to cells for respiration. Lack of iron leads to anemia and a "tired feeling" because the blood is inefficient in carrying oxygen. Obviously, body cells do not work well when lacking in oxygen. Iron comes from red meat, cereals and prune juice.

Trace minerals like copper, zinc, selenium and manganese are needed in very small amounts. Few people need to worry about these. They, too, combine in some obscure metabolic processes left for physiologists to study. They come in drinking water and assorted foods.

A quick question: Do we need more vitamins and minerals? For most people—no. If a balanced diet is being eaten, you and your child will receive enough. If you live a fast paced life with a great deal of activity and stress, one inexpensive multivitamin and mineral supplement can ensure you get all you need. Ask your doctor to be sure.

Food Groups

The nutrients combine to form the basic food groups. The first of the six food groups is the **MILK** group. Milk—the nectar of the cow. It is a staple that can be consumed throughout the life span. Milk contains many of the nutrients we need daily; one of the most notable is calcium. Three eight-ounce servings of lowfat milk per day are necessary for the growing child. Children younger than three years of age should drink whole milk. One cup of milk is approximately equal to one and a half ounces of cheese, one cup of yogurt or two cups of cottage cheese.

The **MEAT** group includes fish, poultry or red meat. Other high protein foods that qualify are cheeses, nuts and beans. The meat group is noted for its large protein availability. Fish and poultry have more protein, ounce for ounce, than any other food outside this group. Two ounces of lean meat is considered one serving. One cup of beans, two ounces of cheese and five tablespoons of peanut butter are also equal to one serving. Children should have two servings each day. For example, if they have one quarter-pound burger, that's all the meat necessary for the entire day.

FRUIT is the next group. Fruit is comprised of a whole realm of items. The most common are apples, oranges and bananas. Each child should have two or more servings daily. A serving is a medium apple, banana or orange.

Children should be encouraged to eat as much fresh fruit as desired. As long as it does not lead to neglect of other food, access to fruit should be unlimited. Snacks should emphasize fruit. Fresh is best. Avoid canned or frozen fruit that has added sugar, salt or preservatives. We are not 100 percent sure whether chemicals and preservatives contribute to behavior problems or hyperactivity, so they are best avoided. The sugar used in processing adds considerable calories to the product. Always have fresh fruit ready for snacking and meals.

VEGETABLES are usually combined with fruit as one category. Both deserve to have some independence, some separate notoriety. Vegetables, like fruit, should be eaten at least twice a day, with unlimited access for meals or snacks. If children want it, they get it any time of the day. Here, too, fresh is best; frozen vegetables are a close second in quality. Avoid highly processed vegetables because of added salt or chemicals. Get a good variety such as lettuce, peas, beans, celery or carrots and wash them carefully. Lightly steam, but don't overcook—too many vitamins are lost. A serving is one cup of raw or half a cup of cooked vegetables or juice.

GRAINS round out the first five groups. Grains include wheat, barley, rice and other grasses that make breads and cereals. Four servings are needed each day. One serving equals one slice of bread or half a cup of cooked grains like pasta, cereal or grits. One full cup of ready-to-eat (low sugar) cereal qualifies as a serving. Grains add fiber and many vitamins and minerals. They are very important for overall nutritional balance.

If your family eats the recommended number of servings from each of the above categories, balance will be brought to your diet. Choose from each of the five basic food groups. Mix different varieties of vegetables, fruit, legumes, grains and lean meats for interest and health. Try to focus on fruit and vegetables because of their filling nature, and *eat only until full*.

One other category exists. It's the **JUNK or OTHER** category. Here dwell the items that didn't get into the first five groups. "Others" are things like soda, condiments, fats, oil or sweets. As far as nutrition is concerned, we all can do with less of these. Most are stripped of their "foodly" identity and don't resemble the grain or vegetable the producer started with. After the extreme processing used in making chips, pretzels, cakes, pies, ice cream or cookies, the loss of nutrition is nearly complete—all you have left is calories. In other words—JUNK! It's not worth eating. As said by one nutrition critic, "It's better to eat the box it came in than to eat the junk food itself."

In small quantities, junk food won't harm the healthy child and may add some variety to life. As I stated earlier in the book, you should never completely avoid something unless you really want to. Don't hook yourself or the family into feeling deprived. Deprivation is the fastest way to foster a desire to have the forbidden fruit. *But please opt to avoid junk as much as possible.* Don't buy it yourself, and watch and see if your children get it at school. (Sometimes schools have junk food machines which get the money intended for lunches. Does yours?) All that is gained in eating junk is extra calories with little or no nutrition. No place is reserved for these foods, if they can be called foods, in nutrition.

Recommended Servings

	Serving Size	*Number Per Day*
Milk	1 cup skim or lowfat milk 1½ ounces of cheese	3
Meat	2 ounces of lean meat fish, poultry 1 cup cooked beans	2
Fruit	1 item such as medium orange, banana, apple	2 or more
Vegetable	1 cup raw, ½ cup cooked	2 or more
Grain	1 cup ready-to-eat cereal 1 slice of bread ½ cup cooked pasta	4
Junk	1 snack per week	

Make a copy of this chart and place it on your refrigerator as a reminder to you and your children.

Menu Planning

Menu planning begins with certain basic guidelines. These are:

• Meals and snacks should be planned in advance. Have a general time that meals and snacks are eaten. Stay as close to those times as possible. Have a morning and afternoon snack and three meals.

• Children should have no set calorie restrictions. We will not worry about how many calories are eaten. Calorie counting is out!

• Meals should not be rushed and, if possible, the child should be rested before eating.

• Unlimited fruits and vegetables should be provided throughout the day as snacks (as long as other foods are not excluded). If a child eats so much fruit that little else is eaten, restrict snacks to two per day. You may draw up a snack sheet so the child can indicate whenever he has a snack. This will keep him aware of his snacking.

• Parents control the types of food presented at meals and snacks. You choose what to eat. Certainly, at times, you should respond to requests if they're deemed reasonable.

• Periodically, new foods should be offered without inducements, bribes or rewards for eating. Eat some yourself and let the child do the same. If he doesn't eat it, that's OK. Maybe the next time he will.

• Food should be presented in small bites, in a colorful way with mild seasoning. Don't go overboard with seasoning, and avoid salt.

• Avoid casseroles and sauces. Young children like to identify food. Don't cover it up or mix together many ingredients.

• **Children should dictate how much and if they eat at each meal. Do not force them to eat!**

Let's stop for a moment because this is the most controversial suggestion in the entire book. What does it mean? Exactly what it says: Children should dictate how much and if they eat. This may be hard for you to swallow. But it is important. It ties in with the beginning of the book when I pointed out how physiological hunger must drive eating behavior. All people have to learn their own body cues that signal fullness. It is more difficult than it sounds.

The only way for them to learn physical hunger is to let your children start and stop themselves. You must inform each child about proper nutrition. You must educate him about food and eating. But ultimately the child must decide to eat or not. If you force him to eat, he forms a reliance on outside controls. Unfortunately, in this manner children do not learn adequate personal control. You do it for them. That does not work for the long term unless you plan to do it for the rest of their lives. Likewise, your control can induce resentment and actually cause your children to eat more, defeating any attempts to help.

Experience will teach adequate control. You help guide the process of discovery by getting the child to focus on fullness, by increasing enjoyment and influencing proper food selection.

It will take time to get used to this step. Allow for it. Guide toward good, sound nutrition. But the child is the one with the "yea" or "nay" to eating. Remember the old proverb, "You can lead a kid to spinach but you can't make him eat it." (Or was that a horse to water?) At any rate, DON'T FORCE EATING.

Refer back to the observation sheet on Food Selection in Chapter Two. How do the Favorite Foods stack up to being balanced? Are the first five food categories well represented? What changes do you need to make?

Most of you are going to dictate a new emphasis on fruit, vegetables and grains. Cultivation of taste based on a wide range of foods is the first step. Keep unlimited access to fresh fruit and vegetables while sticking to a base of four ounces of lean meat, fish or poultry and three glasses of lowfat milk per day. You virtually have free reign over what to have and prepare. For the most part, you will continue eating much of what you had before—only less. You do not have to make radical dietary changes. Here are some other ideas:

Milk

You should have three eight-ounce glasses per day. One trick is to use nonfat dry milk and put in 30 percent more powder—lots of protein and calcium. Serve well chilled. Or substitute one glass for one cup of yogurt. Mix in some fruit for dessert. It also tastes good frozen. Or try one and a half ounces of cheese. Try different varieties. It makes a good snack or dessert. Melt some over vegetables or in a sandwich.

Meat

Children need two two-ounce servings (4 oz. total). Beef should be lean with all visible fat removed. Broil, roast, or bake.

Allow fat to drip away from the meat and discard. If you eat hamburger, get the leanest possible. It ends up being cheaper, as it doesn't all cook away. With pork remove all visible fat and roast. For poultry, remove the skin and all visible fat. Broil, roast or bake. Avoid frying. Fish is good anytime, baked or broiled. Use lemon and spices. Don't use butter on it. Tuna fish sandwiches are easy for lunch. Remember, one can (6 oz.) is three servings. Use lowfat mayonnaise. Shellfish is not as high in cholesterol as was once thought and is a nice treat once in a while. Boil, bake or roast. No deep frying! Two medium eggs are a single serving. With the controversy surrounding cholesterol, eggs are best eaten in moderation. Stick to three or four egg yokes per week. (The yolk has all the cholesterol.) Combine the whites of two eggs as one serving and discard the yoke to avoid excess cholesterol.

Nuts

Two ounces equal one meat serving. Nuts have a good amount of protein but are a little heavy on the fat content—a nice taste treat on occasions. Get the unsalted varieties. Try almonds, brazils, cashews, filberts, pecans, pine nuts, pistachios and walnuts.

Fruit

Two servings per day is the *minimum*. One medium fruit equals a serving. One cup of berries is a serving. Get fresh or frozen. Avoid canned or frozen fruit that has added sugar; the label should say "packed in its own juice." Try apples, apricots, bananas, blackberries, blueberries, cherries, dates, figs, grapefruit, grapes, melons, nectarines, oranges, pears, pineapple, plums, raspberries, strawberries, tangelos and tangerines. Often, some unusual fruits come into season. Check the produce section. You may see kiwi fruit, mangos and papayas, Try them out—a little titillation for tired taste buds.

Vegetables

You should have two servings per day (one serving = one cup raw or half a cup cooked). Buy fresh or frozen. Canning adds salt as a preservative. Check the label. Steaming retains the vitamins. If boiling, use as little water as possible. Don't let the vitamins wash away during cooking. Also, learn about stir-frying in a wok; or use the microwave with a little water to steam vegetables. Keep them crispy. Do not over-cook! Try artichokes, asparagus, beets, broccoli, brussel sprouts, cabbage, carrots, cauliflower, celery, corn, eggplant, green beans, jicama, kale, lettuce, mushrooms, onions, peas, potatoes, radishes, spinach, sprouts, squash, turnips, watercress and beans. Beans come in many varieties as do many of the other vegetables. One cup of cooked beans is equal to one meat serving. See what you can find in your grocery store or market.

Grains

Everyone should have four servings of grains per day. One serving equals one slice of bread, half a cup cooked cereal or pasta, or one cup ready-to-eat cereal. Try breads of many varieties; avoid bleached white flour. Buy whole wheat or whole grain breads; but it *must* say 100% Whole Grain. Read the ingredients! Also try whole grains, such as barley, millet, rice, cereal, pasta, buckwheat or flours. Try each grain in cereals and soups, or as a side dish.

For more information on how to prepare foods, go to your local library or book store and pick up a cookbook on using fresh fruit, vegetables and lean meats. Look for new ideas and recipes in magazines or obtain them from family or friends. Be creative.

Plan your meals by making selections from each of the five categories. Work for balance with servings from each food group every day. See that each family member has an opportunity to select from all food groups to obtain balanced meals.

Snacks

Snacks are a must. But build snacks that will deliver a punch and not a paunch. Snacks can be and should be nutritious. Try peanut butter on whole grain crackers, celery, apples or other fruit. Tastes good!

Or try vegetable or fruit juices blended with whole fruit and ice. A great summer treat. If you choose canned juices, watch out for salt or sugar! Get no-calorie flavored mineral waters. Many children like to drink them as a soda substitute or mix them with fruit juices for a low-calorie drink. Mix skim milk with fruit in a blender. Yum!

Stuff the refrigerator full of vegetables. Prepare them in advance for easy access. Buy a large jar and fill it with celery, carrots and a little water—a quick snack.

An unlimited supply of fresh fruit is excellent for snacks. Don't skimp on the fruit. Buy something new each week. Dried fruit is a nice change with highly concentrated nutrition.

Try popcorn without butter and salt. Try topping with grated Parmesan or cheddar cheese, garlic or onion powder. Add shelled nuts and seeds, raisins or parsley. If the family likes spicy food, try sprinkling on some crushed or powdered red and black pepper, hot pepper sauce or anything else you discover in the spice rack.

Buy sunflower seeds, peanuts (which are legumes rather than nuts) or other nuts. Get them in the shell, as they take longer to eat and it's more fun. Varieties of nuts abound, but watch for added salt.

Try freezing some fruit juice in a plastic glass with a stick in it. Tastes better than popsicles! Freeze yogurt with fresh fruit mixed in—a good ice cream substitute.

Other snacks you like:

1. _____
2. _____

Sample Menu

Breakfast
1 oz. shredded wheat
1 cup lowfat milk
1 slice 100% whole wheat toast
1 pat of margarine
8 oz. orange juice

Lunch
tuna sandwich (2 oz. tuna, 2 slices whole wheat bread, 1 tbsp. lowfat mayonnaise)
1 cup low sodium tomato soup
1 cup pineapple packed in its own juice
mineral water

Dinner
2 oz. chicken with skin removed
½ cup steamed green beans
½ cup oven baked french fries
1 cup lowfat milk
1 cup bananas and cherries topped with ½ oz. crushed pecans

Morning Snack (Optional)
apple or orange mineral water*

Afternoon Snack
1 cup yogurt mixed with fresh strawberries
mineral water

Evening Snack
2 cups unbuttered popcorn with 1 oz. unsalted nuts mixed in
mineral water

Provides:
Milk — 3 servings (milk, yogurt)
Meat — 2½ servings (tuna, chicken, nuts)
Grains — 4 servings (cereal, bread)
Vegetables — 4 servings (soup, beans, fries, popcorn)
Fruit — 4 servings (orange juice, pineapple, fresh fruit)

*Mineral water — A variety of flavored water products are available. They have a carbonation zing like soda but usually have no zap from calories. These are a good drink substitute for soda and can be mixed with juices for a new taste treat.

Shopping List

Making lists will help avoid impulse buying. First, take time to think about next week's meals. When you have a basic idea as to what to prepare, including snacks, make a list of the foods necessary for the menu. Second, eat before you shop. If you are not hungry when shopping, you are less likely to pick up items that aren't needed.

Most of all, stick to the list! Do not buy junk. Stay away from those rows of magnetic munchies that jump into unsuspecting carts. If junk isn't in the house, it will not be tempting the kids. Don't buy chips except for an occasional bag of one of the low-salt varieties. Substitute whole wheat crackers or popcorn. Avoid buying soda (get juice or flavored mineral water), cookies (try low-sugar granola), cakes (try fruit) or pie (yogurt with fresh fruit). Find substitutes for many of your family's traditional junk foods. Use your imagination.

Labels

Labels are written with the major ingredients first. Lesser-used ingredients come later, depending on how much of each is inside the box or can. The rule of thumb is: If sugar, salt or oils are the first three ingredients of a product, avoid it. The item is mostly junk. Labels must also provide the following information:

1. Size of a serving.
2. Number of servings in the package.
3. Number of calories in a serving.
4. Grams of protein, fat and carbohydrates in a serving.
5. The percentage or the Recommended Daily Allowance (RDA) in one serving of vitamins A, C, B1, B2, niacin, calcium, iron and protein. The RDA is the expected amount of the nutrients needed by the average healthy individual. Use the RDA as a guideline as to the product's nutritional value.

Read the label carefully. It will tell you how much nutrition you are getting for your money. Shop and compare the RDAs. Find the best deal and stick with it. Likewise, avoid anything that has a large amount of salt, sugar or ingredients you cannot pronounce. You will all be healthier for it.

Storage

Most foods should be stored away, out of sight. This is especially true for the foods you do not want the child to get into. If you have to buy some junk food, keep it in the most obscure cabinet in the kitchen. Alternatively, fruit and vegetables should be readily accessible. Foods with good nutritional content should be right out front in the refrigerator, all ready to be eaten. And *no* candy dishes around the house!

If you must buy junk food, try to get items requiring preparation time. The longer it takes to prepare a snack, the less likely it will be eaten. That's why fruit should be ready to eat on a moment's notice. The fastest snack is usually the one that is eaten first.

Next, leftovers can be a problem. A child should not be forced to eat everything on his plate. Thus, leftovers will occur. Some parents think it is a sin to throw away food. I think it is a sin to become overfat. Leftovers *can* be discarded. If you feel guilty about getting rid of food because someone is starving in Africa, please place all leftovers in a storage container and ship them overseas.

Short of transoceanic shipments of leftovers, place all foods in containers that can't be seen through. Then freeze it for another time. Don't leave leftovers in the refrigerator to be nibbled on. If you can't get to it easily, neither can your child. Out of sight, out of mouth.

Food Selection Game

The Food Selection Game is one of the family structured conversations you can use at dinner time. As you remember from the chapter on Head Stuff, structured conversation can enhance family interaction. Learning is also a benefit of the process. Teaching nutrition is one of the best table activities.

This game can take many forms. First, you can have the children choose what they want to eat from the foods you have cooked. Have them select what and how much they would like to eat. While they make selections, ask what category the food comes from. By questioning, you teach them to put together a plate with meat, vegetables and fruit. Quiz them on the food taken and what amounts are needed for proper balance.

Once the basic categories are known, quizzes can occur at the table. For example, someone names a food. Other family members guess its category. The person who answers correctly goes next. Start with today's table foods. Next, name other foods not on the table. The person who answers gets a point. Points are tallied and rewards are given in whatever way you choose.

Another game to be played away from the table to teach identification of food categories is to make playing cards with pictures of food. This is similar to flash-cards that are used in arithmetic. Show the card to the child and he guesses the category. Make up a reward system using verbal praise and little trinkets for good work. The child can also make collages of the food categories to help learn about eating. Any craft can be used to help him understand nutrition. Let that creativity blossom!

What types of games or projects can you think of?

Together, some or all of these tactics can combine to give good nutrition with even better weight control.

Finally, Back to Susan, Bill, Jimmy and John

Susan and Bill had to break out of their traditional Midwest meal doldrums. The parents recognized that they ate far too much meat and potatoes. Meat is high in protein but also very high in fat. Potatoes are fine vegetables. The potato, per se, was not the culprit in their children's overfatness. The two villains were what was put on the potatoes and how the potatoes were cooked. Plenty of fat was in those spuds. Sour cream was piled high on baked potatoes and oil loaded those home fries. This was far too much fat in the diet of a family with a history of heart disease.

Susan started to introduce some new foods. Resistance cropped up quickly. She did not fight with the boys or force them to eat. Susan only modeled eating new things. She ate as the boys looked on. Bill tried the new dishes, too. Seeing their father leading, the boys tried an occasional dish.

To avoid starting too quickly, Susan had some familiar foods available. Over time, she slowly introduced more new dishes. Soon, half of the items in the meals were new dishes she had created. The boys joined in to eat some of each.

After six weeks of the new foods, Susan started to decrease the amount of meat at the table. She used more beans and lentils. Soup became a more prominent item on the menu. It was easy to put together in the morning and let cook all day in the crockpot. The boys liked soup and readily ate it.

Next, Susan served a greater variety of vegetables in a raw or lightly cooked state. The boys could use their fingers to eat them and they had more fun eating "rabbit food." Despite their joking, everyone was eating.

Meals seemed to be going well. The family was eating many more vegetables and starting to have fruit for dessert. Major resistance from the boys was waning. Susan was relieved to find the whole family changing their mealtime eating habits and no one had starved to death in the meantime. In addition, the family chose to eat more at home and stayed away from fast food as much as possible. Overall, they found they did not miss it except for Jimmy wailing about his fries. A trip to the "Golden Insteps" still occurred once in a while for variety.

But as meals went well, a tough part was still to come. Snacking had to change.

Chips and popcorn ruled the snacking scene. The boys liked popcorn with lots of butter on top. But the butter brought in major calories (and overfatness). Popcorn itself was a good snack. Removing the butter, they had something that could be eaten to their coronary arteries' content. Susan tried some new toppings to see if the boys would eat it. A few were acceptable.

Cheese was a good alternative; so was hot sauce. They also tried other spices on the popcorn. Susan stocked up and they tried new ones each week. Popcorn was disappearing and the young ones were happy. The good thing was the popcorn was disappearing with far fewer calories than before. It was a much healthier snack without so much butter.

Popcorn was substituted for the majority of the fried snacks. Earlier, the boys had eaten massive quantities of chips. Susan attempted to limit snacking to popcorn as much as possible. She bought a hot air popper and used no oil in the preparation. A few more calories fell by the wayside rather than on to the backside.

To accompany the popcorn and occasional chips, Susan started making juice slushes. She would partially freeze some fruit juice and put it in a glass. The boys would stir it up and chug it down. It was very refreshing and a healthy alternative to drinking so much soda.

The family was coming to the conclusion that eating habits could change without sacrificing all fun and flavor. Food selections were changing. In conjunction with increased exercise, weight gains were on the downturn. The boys slowed their girth growth to a much more reasonable level for their ages. Food costs were down and morale had not suffered. It was working.

Summary

After reading this chapter you may feel that some of your family's food habits are in need of further revision. To ensure proper nutrition, you must focus on the food groups and attempt to include each in its recommended proportion. It takes time but brings about an abundance of health over the years. Teach your child the right foods to eat. Begin with your current menu. What are:

- Some foods to limit

- Some foods to add

- Snacks to be limited

- Snacks to be added

Chapter Six

Unstuff: Maintaining Control

Maintenance comes by periodically reviewing your family's habits.

•

Habits become life styles after consistent practice.

•

Changes continue by rewarding good habits.

•

Keep setting realistic goals. Reward your child when goals are attained.

•

Get support from groups: the YMCA/YWCA, schools or health clubs.

•

Start your own Kid's STUFF group. Work with others who are dealing with the problem.

•

Keep weight in its place. Don't let it dominate your child's life.

•

The best of luck (and hard work) to you all!

———————

A journey of a thousand miles
begins with one step.
— Old Chinese Proverb

Anyone can change. It is a matter of going from one place to another. The real question is: will they stay or return to the site from whence they came?

As in moving, to take up a new, permanent residence requires planning and forethought. Otherwise, you cannot establish yourself. Maintenance of weight control requires planning and vigilance to ensure desired changes become a part of life. Breaking old habits is like a long journey. One must take numerous steps to finish. These steps take effort and willingness.

To ensure habits have been firmly established, the family must monitor themselves periodically. After about two to six months of following the specifics of the program, most families evolve techniques into everyday habits. It takes time. Remember the first time on a bike? You concentrated very hard to keep balanced. It took a while to get comfortable. After practicing, it was easy. You didn't have to think about balance; riding became instinctive. The same will occur with this program.

Children need *at least* two months of practice to "balance" the basics. As the habits become natural, a feeling of comfort arises. Children are very adaptable. They can learn quickly, but must be reminded of goals on occasion. Forgetfulness does happen; sometimes attention is short. Therefore review is a very necessary part of the program.

Children must continue to apply techniques until performance becomes as easy as riding a bike. The best insurance for continued change is to review tactics by evaluation. One way to review is to fill out the assessment forms in Chapter Two, just as if you were first starting. Then you ask the questions: Are you still using good eating habits, getting exercise and selecting good food? Is anything not being followed as before? Check it out.

If there are problems, go back to the section of the book that pertains to the habits in question. Reread. You may go through part or all of the program again. It will be easier the second time. Change will be quicker, as you are not starting from scratch. But recognize why a restart is necessary and avoid those pitfalls in the future.

Most families will need this periodic review to maintain major change. You may even expect to review the program at specific intervals. A typical plan would be to review changes at three-, six-, and/or twelve-month intervals. If change has been firmly established, the review time will be short and will help keep habits sharp. If you find positive consistency between reviews, the family is doing well. If problems are found, take as much time as necessary to get back on track. No time constraints truly exist. This program is for life.

All along, it has been presumed that all adults in the household agree that change is necessary. An atmosphere of family support is vital. Lack of caring, attention or indifference to the program will bring about its demise. Nothing will change, nothing will improve. In fact, further family problems may befall the unwary couple.

Lack of working together between spouses is especially devastating. It signals fundamental problems in the marital relationship—a tough thing to think about. Do you have marital concerns? Don't let the children suffer from relationship problems. If this is occurring, such as when the parents can't agree on how to use this program, you will want to read about resistance in the next chapter.

As starting slow has been a virtue, it is a virtue in review. Always begin with small goals. Set the priorities with simple changes so that you can ensure some success at first. Larger goals come later. Create early victories.

Define goals clearly. Do you want eating, exercise or food selection habits to change? How are you going to do it? Review your tactics. Know what you are after.

Much of what is in this book is basic problem-solving. So, at any time, you can foster change in this way, regardless of the problem at hand. Remember, the basic steps in good problem-solving are:

- Define the problem. What is wrong?
- How, when, and why does it happen?
- What have you done to change it before?
- What are other solutions and consequences?
- Try a new solution.
- Did it work? What was the outcome?

Follow your tactics to a final solution. Break down problems into steps. Piece the steps together. Gather alternatives to attack the problem. See which options bring viable solutions. Then always evaluate your outcomes.

In addition, the major focus should be on the positives. Remember to reinforce good behavior. Avoid anger, frustration and disgust to the greatest extent that is humanly possible. Look at ways of making the positive changes overwhelm the negative. Growth occurs in a well fertilized field. Optimal expression can be obtained with the right growth material. There is, however, a difference between being fertilized and being dumped on.

As change most readily occurs with praise, criticism will surely destroy the esteem of the child. Since overfatness has its own pain, don't do anything that will chip away at self-esteem. Support as much as possible. Talk and play together. Make sure the child knows he is worthwhile. He most certainly is!

Supporting the esteem of the child is necessary to foster behavior changes with lasting meaning. Punishment will take away from esteem, causing it to falter. Learning results from a supportive environment. Eventually the child can even teach others in a supportive way. Control will flourish; change is sustained.

Sustenance also comes from having a wide variety of resources. For example, starting a KID S.T.U.F.F. GROUP will aid in long-term control. Group support is a powerful way of creating motivation and adherence. Schools, the YMCA/YWCA or others may help to create a group that will adopt this type of a program. If not, they certainly have their own style of groups and exercise classes. Take advantage of groups in any way possible. From monitoring to maintenance, groups can help to make changes as well as be stable ground for support. Since many overfat children lack esteem, a group can provide considerable support and show he is not alone.

Another issue is that of the single parent. Single parents have special needs. Rearing a child alone is especially difficult. It may seem overwhelming to start a program on your own—many obligations are already lined up. A group can help combat this dilemma. Don't take everything on yourself unless you can devote the time. Get help. Otherwise, you may feel more frustrated than before.

For everyone concerned, do what you can. Put all resources at your disposal. See what is available in the community. Give your family the best chance possible in the prevention of overfatness. Weight control will serve the whole family an entire lifetime.

What tactics do you need to employ to maintain good habits?

Dates for reviewing program: Three months_____

   Six months_____One year_____

Groups I can contact are:_____

Is there anything else I need to consider?_____

Chapter Seven

Tough Stuff: Questions From Parents

In this chapter, I will present some of the most interesting and important questions asked in weight control groups. The questions may address some of your own concerns. For your convenience, the subject of each question is highlighted for quick reference. Related information on the subject may be obtained by referring to any capitalized words contained in the answer.

The questions are meant to give further information. This is not, however, an attempt to offer medical or psychological advice. If you have specific questions about your child, go to your pediatrician, family doctor or psychologist.

My child uses all his allowance to buy candy and other junk foods. Also, he eats at times without my knowing it. What can I do to get him to stop?

Lack of cooperation with young children happens occasionally. They have not yet learned how to delay gratification. Many will indulge in a covert snack. But when a child spends his entire allowance on candy or is eating heavily when parents are absent, this is not acceptable. It is a sign of RESISTANCE that must be approached with understanding and firmness.

To begin with, parents must sit down with the child and tell him directly that to use all his money on junk food is not healthy and is not acceptable to you. Just as you would not let him spend his money on drugs, he isn't to spend it all on food. Ask him if he understands that buying a great deal of candy is contrary to the program and unhealthy. Discuss it. Why does he do it? What can you do to help him with it? Suggest a contract, with the child helping to write the terms. Then write a contract stating that allowance money will only be used for non-food items. Some flexibility must be included. For example, one or two snacks per week is acceptable as long as he gets your permission first. That helps to keep the child from seeking the "forbidden fruit."

In addition, you may suggest taking a walk after eating snacks or walking to the store when a snack is desired. Don't keep snacks in the house. Walking to the store will burn calories. But remember — do not make this seem like punishment. Make it time for the two of you to talk and be close.

Of course many children are not mature enough to make contracts work. Suzie, age eight, could not follow her contract consistently, so her parents decided they would supervise allowances. Suzie's parents would accompany her to the store and give Suzie her weekly allowance. Suzie was restricted to the purchase of non-foods. She could buy clothes, toys or anything else she wanted. If she did not spend all her money, Mom would hold the balance until the next shopping trip.

Nathan, 13, was more independent than Suzie. He presented additional problems for supervision as his usual allowance payment led to a binge on hamburgers and fries when out with his friends. One way to decrease the excessive eating was to have his father split Nathan's allowance into smaller, equal parts. Nathan could not buy a complete meal with that much money. His father was flexible though: If Nathan planned to go to a movie, he would get more money as needed. However, if Nathan tried to save up his money for another binge, he would miss out on activities with friends. Much of the excessive eating was reduced.

The next step to take when your child is eating heavily behind your back and is still difficult to control is to make a contract with the child to receive rewards when he maintains his weight. If the scale doesn't move—reward. Give an important reward such as time, money or a trinket. A reward can bring a great deal of covert eating under control if it is powerful enough. (As the child continues to grow, make some allowances for increasing weight.)

Furthermore, if rewards fail, you may move toward sanctions for continued excessive weight gain. Do this as a last resort. For instance, take away allowances for gaining weight due to spending on food. Reward if he doesn't gain; sanction if he does. You can take away other rewarding items if the child continues to eat covertly and gain excessively. Again, it is always best to reward first. Then take away valued activities or possessions as weight increases. As weight stabilizes, return lost privileges quickly.

Eventually, of course, the child will grow and normally gain weight. But depending on the amount of bodyfat, many children will grow a number of inches before they need gain further weight. Ask your physician for guidance on growth patterns.

If none of this works for you, you should consult a psychologist or other mental health professional trained in family therapy or eating disorders. Further attempts at control will only frustrate the family. Never use put-downs or negative remarks to "shame" the child into losing weight or stopping any behavior. It won't work and could contribute to the formation of an eating disorder.

What is anorexia nervosa?

Anorexia is a psychological syndrome where a person becomes very fearful of gaining weight. It mostly affects adolescent and college-age women. Due to striving for a "perfect figure," dieting and exercise become excessive. The preoccupation with overfatness worsens. Body image becomes distorted and anorexics "feel fat" even though weight is average or below normal. As eating substantially decreases, metabolic changes occur. Women may stop having menstrual periods and become malnourished. Once 25 percent of original bodyweight is lost and they refuse to maintain a normal weight, a diagnosis of anorexia nervosa may be rendered.

It must be emphasized that this is a syndrome that requires professional help. Ten to 15 percent of anorexics die. Don't try to treat it on your own or force the adolescent to eat. It may get worse. Anorexics often hide weight losses from parents. If you suspect your adolescent is very underweight, may have induced VOMITING or refuses to eat, you may want to talk to your doctor or a psychologist who has experience in treating eating disorders. Don't wait. A life could depend on it.

The school counselor says my child is anxious. What is anxiety?

Anxiety is a feeling of dread or apprehension about the future. The dread may or may not have a specific cause. Over time, as fears continue, the child may have physical symptoms or complain of being "sick" when no medical problems can be found.

Children have many fears. If your child appears unusually sensitive, try to find out what is bothering him. Much of childhood anxiety is situational. It is temporary and is in response to some stressor. Spend some time talking. What can you do together to remove that stress? Engaging in some sort of play or walks helps to diffuse some of the physical feelings of anxiety. If the problem persists, seek professional help.

Behavior modification sounds extreme. What is it?

Behavior modification or B-mod has obtained a bad reputation. It evokes images of shocking people so they salivate to the sound of a dog barking. All it really is, is a generic term for a number of techniques to change behavior. B-mod is based in behavioral theory. The term "behavior therapy" has been substituted in most instances today. It only refers to changing habits and behavior. It is no more specific than that.

What is binge eating and what is it associated with?

Overeating is common at times. Binge eating, however, is an extreme form of overeating where a person may eat thousands of calories at a single sitting. Some may eat a whole gallon of ice cream, a box of chocolates and several bags of cookies at once. Obviously, the person is in acute discomfort afterwards.

Often, vomiting will be induced to get rid of the food and avoid weight gain. This happens in ANOREXIA NERVOSA but is most often associated with BULIMIA.

Binge eating may be a reaction to stress. People use food to bury a vast array of feelings. It is a red flag that something is very wrong. Due to the physical and psychological problems that arise from binge eating, professional help must be sought if it continues for more than two days or recurs periodically.

What is bulimia?

Bulimia is a psychological syndrome where the adolescent or adult eats large amounts of food. She may eat so much that pain is experienced, then vomit or use laxatives to get rid of the food to avoid weight gain. She is caught between a tremendous urge to eat and stay slim at the same time.

The victim knows it is a problem but cannot stop. Often, depression is very prominent in her life. She feels out of control. Eating may temporarily defeat feelings of depression or other discomfort. But soon the cycle of bingeing and purging continues.

Bulimia arises with many attempts to lose weight by very restrictive diets and heavy exercise. When diet and exercise fail to give the desired figure, or when feelings of deprivation arise, bulimics resort to the use of vomiting and laxatives after eating excessively. Even though purging rids most of the calories, the bulimic absorbs enough food to be close to normal weight. In contrast, anorexics tend to look very thin.

Typically, as with ANOREXIA NERVOSA, the person feels worthless and is very fearful of being discovered. Secretiveness pervades her life. Few friends ever suspect a problem.

We don't know how often it occurs. It tends to be very common in college coeds who like to eat but wish to stay thin. Cultural obsession with slim female figures plays a part in the beginnings of anorexia and bulimia.

Some anorexics will also binge and purge. A combination of anorexia and bulimia is common. Both bulimia and anorexia can lead to death. Physical problems eventually arise from vomiting. Tooth decay occurs due to stomach acid, metabolic imbalance surfaces because of the loss of acids, and torn abdominal muscles occur via the force of vomiting.

Bulimia is a disorder that needs prompt professional help. The longer one waits, the harder it is to stop. The way to avoid anorexia or bulimia is to teach proper weight management skills at an early age. Don't let your family members get involved with dogmatic diets, extreme exercise or frivolous fads.

Are physicians now taking blood pressure in children more seriously?

Yes. Pediatricians are now monitoring blood pressure in children more intently. It is still somewhat rare to find high blood pressure in kids. It is, however, being found. Treatment with diet and exercise will help most children. Dumping the salt shaker out the window helps, too.

You should monitor your child's blood pressure via your doctor. Spaces on the assessment forms in Chapter Two are available for that purpose. Ask your pediatrician for more details about what to do for your child to monitor blood pressure.

Why don't you count calories in your program?

Children should never be forced to count calories. They should be taught the nutritional value and categories of food. Counting calories is an unnatural way of weight control. It is tedious and time consuming.

The person of average weight does not count calories. I want children to learn naturally about how much food they need on a daily basis. That knowledge comes through guided trial and error. With your help, they see how much to eat and how it impacts on weight.

This program has the older child keep a food log. He can write down what was eaten. Once a serving size is well understood, he can monitor himself and keep fairly accurate records. Then the parent has a basic idea as to what the child is eating when away from home.

The ultimate quest is to get children to *think* as average weight people *think*. They naturally know how much to eat and when they feel full. Your child needs to learn the same skill. It will take time, but will provide for internal controls from the child, rather than external controls from the parent. And since you cannot and should not control every aspect of his life, he must learn to do it.

My boy and I seem to fight over food often. What do I do?

This is a tough question. The answer may come down to improving communication. Parents often will get caught in a challenge and power struggle situation. Rather than trying to force the child to eat, it is best to try to clarify the communication going on.

Reflect back to the child what you think he is saying rather than ordering him to eat. When he says, "I won't eat this!" you respond, "Oh, you don't like this type of food?" "Yes, it doesn't taste good." "What would you rather have?" And so on. To order your child to eat would lead to a "Yes, you will"/"No, I won't" battle. By trying to clarify what the child is saying, you can avoid the challenge and see if the child has some legitimate concerns. If so, you may change your view. If it is an important issue and a conflict develops, see what to do in TIME OUT.

I found a bunch of food under my daughter's bed. What does this mean?

HOARDING. Sometimes kids are just messy. They like to have some sort of snack. However, keeping food under the bed is not allowed. Remember, you want to restrict eating to certain places as much as possible. Food should not be kept in the bedroom.

In extreme cases of hoarding, it may be a clue that other problems are brewing. For instance, individuals displaying ANOREXIA NERVOSA will hide food they don't eat. That way, parents think they are eating, when in fact, they are not. Likewise, in BULIMIA people will stockpile food for a binge. This is a very deliberate action in these cases. In this specific instance, it is hard to say why the food is under the bed. Don't overreact. Talk to the child and see what may be going on.

How do you cope with holidays?

Holidays are special times that invite overeating. It is best to have a wide variety of foods and take a *sampling* of many things. Just have fun. Don't be overly restrictive.

Let the child prepare his own plate. Everyone should try to remember to eat moderately. Drinking a glass of water prior to eating will help to bring on feelings of fullness. Review and talk about good habits prior to eating—but don't nag! Once the meal is over, food should be put away to avoid nibbling. Further, a walk may aid digestion and help to get away from excess food.

Before, during and after the holidays increase exercise to compensate for the extra eating. Recognize that more eating goes on during these times. It's normal. No guilt, no pain. Work it off together to get *no* gain.

My in-laws and neighbors will give candy to the kids. How can I get them to stop?

Talk to them directly. Don't beat around the bush. Tell them that you are engaging in a weight control program. You appreciate that they are so caring as to give candy. However, you would like them to do it differently. Could they suggest an alternative—praise the child or give him a little trinket instead of candy? A fine suggestion. Maybe you could engage the in-laws' help in other ways. Agree on an alternative and stick to it.

Do not dictate to them but see how you can engage their help in weight control. Most adults would be happy to help. Suggest alternatives and agree together. If they still don't comply, try to figure out why. Is there a power struggle or is it that they can't say "NO" to the child? Try to understand what is going on. Keep communication lines open.

My child will only eat a limited variety of foods. What do I do?

Children will limit types of foods for many reasons. At different stages this is normal. Don't try to force them to eat more. Let them explore at their own pace. However, when some have become overly restrictive for more than three months, action should be taken. First, see your pediatrician for advice. Make sure there are no physical problems. Second, if all is well, start a brief change in program.

Try this approach: Have a favorite food ready to eat with a number of alternate or new foods. Give one of the alternate foods. Praise the child if he takes it. If he won't, allow him to have some of the favorite food. Don't say *anything*.

Again, try the alternate. Don't bribe. If he does take the new food, give profuse praise and allow him to have some more of the preferred food. Use his favorite food as reinforcement for eating something new.

Give another bite of the new food. Continue to praise whenever it is taken. *Ignore anything else he does.* Do not beg, plead, threaten or cajole. As soon as he takes a bite, let him know that's good.

Praise when he takes the new food but don't punish for noncompliance. Ignore him momentarily when he is not eating the new food. If he totally refuses to eat anything new, be very matter-of-fact and allow him to eat more of the favorite food. Once having eaten adequate calories, immediately leave the table and withdraw attention for three to five minutes. Then resume normal table cleanup activities.

Try this for several days. Make other new foods available. Keep up praising when new foods are taken. Ignore behavior when not eating the new, although you should respond normally to questions or non-disruptive table talk. If he takes a new food, immediately verbally reward him and give a hug.

Over several weeks, as he starts to take more of the new foods, slowly wean him away from so much attention for eating new foods. Once in a while, reward him for eating them. Start with every other bite; then every third and so on. Continue to give periodic attention when new and varied foods are eaten.

Start from the beginning if he slips back.

Should this not work and the child is failing to thrive, not growing or seemingly ill, consult professional help.

When my son was a year-and-a-half old he ate dirt and other non-foods. Is that unusual?

PICA. Rare, but not necessarily unusual. We do not know a great deal about pica. It seems to occur in one-to-two-year-olds who may have an iron deficiency. Youngsters will eat a variety of non-nutritive substances. It becomes a serious problem when they eat glass or lead based paints. For most children, this behavior stops on its own shortly after age two. If it continues beyond, get an opinion from your pediatrician as to your child's iron level and nutritional status.

Are school physical education classes helpful?

Yes. All children who are physically able should take these classes at school. It is a way of gaining exposure to different sports and activities. Be sure, however, that it is a positive experience with a variety of games that your child can engage in. Competent supervision must be provided. P.E. is one of the few times your child can play and learn about exercise all at the same time.

The kids seem to constantly poke around in the kitchen. How can we cut down on this?

PROWLING AND GRAZING. All of us, at times, graze around the kitchen like cattle looking for a patch of grass. It is often a sign of boredom or anxiety. If it is, your child must find other ways of relieving those feelings. Give a snack if you have not already done so. If snacks are over for the day, see if activity will keep them busy. Take a walk if possible. Do something physical to burn up that energy. Have a supply of games or other activities. See what activities you can come up with. Doing nothing guarantees something is about to be eaten.

What about punishment?

Punishment plays no part in this program. Behavior change is consistently better and longer lasting when positive reinforcement is used. Reward good behavior. The child knows exactly what behavior is acceptable, rather than what you don't want.

Punishment is distasteful for the parent and has the emotional side effect of distancing the child from people. The child knows he has done wrong but may not know what to do right. Don't use punishment, but discipline with the TIME OUT procedures explained later in this chapter.

What are some reinforcements we should use?

Praise is the number one source of reinforcement or reward. Telling the children exactly what they did and why that was good is very important. Get their attention. Say it. Then pat on the back and hug. Still, other reinforcers are having time to play together, to take a walk or to do some other activity. For example, an extra half an hour of playtime with the parent can be won by consistent slow eating.

When using attention to reinforce the child, any attention given should be above and beyond what he normally gets. Give *more* time together when he does well. Otherwise, you risk the child feeling rejected if he doesn't meet the reward requirements. Don't take time away from your child except during TIME OUT. Always give more time whenever he works hard on the program.

To keep track of consistency give stars. A specific number of stars gets an amount of parent time. Stars can also be redeemed for other things such as a trip to the movies, library or pool. Rewards such as a table setting, running shoes or exercise equipment can be used, also.

Determine in advance what you are going to give, how much and for what behavior. Be very specific! Your family values must be taken into account to determine rewards. But, believe me, praise and adult attention are the most powerful.

My family won't cooperate. What do I do?

RESISTANCE.

1. *Spouse.* When a spouse will not cooperate, a signal is being sent out. The signal is that big communication problems are underlying the relationship. This must be remedied before setting out on *any* program. It is important for the parents to work out their differences beforehand and not dump their conflict on the child.

Parents must guard against making the child the object of their dispute. Sometimes parents focus on the children's problems to avoid their own. Everyone loses when that happens. Sabotage is an indicator of unspoken conflict. If you cannot agree after sitting down and discussing it, marital therapy may be necessary. See a counselor.

2. *Child.* Some resistance is normal. If bad habits have become firmly entrenched, change cannot happen overnight. It will take time to relearn new habits. Resistance arises from the propensity for us all to want to keep things the same, even if it would benefit us to do otherwise.

To minimize resistance you must go slowly in your efforts to change. Talk about what you are going to do. Proceed slowly but firmly. A family is not a democratic state. You are the head and must take charge. Resistance will fade with time if you are supportive toward the child and both parents are consistent with the program. Support the child's dignity; children are only human. Treat them as if they are very important people. *They are.*

Should resistance remain firmly embedded in the family, look at how everything is being presented. Make sure it is positive and a joint effort. Do not single out the overfat child. He may feel put on the spot, resentful. Cooperation can't be garnered under these circumstances. Family effort is what this is all about. *It's not any one person's problem.*

Change what you have the most control over. Take easy steps first. Food selection is almost entirely up to the shopping parent. Begin here if you encounter blatant resistance. Present new dishes and let the family decide if they are going to eat or not. They will come around. As they do, move on to other parts of the program.

I heard of a very young child that gained very little weight and was throwing up. What was going on?

Barring any medical problem, the child was experiencing RUMINATION DISORDER. A rare phenomenon called rumination occurs in children three months to one year of age. They fail to gain weight because they throw up. We are not quite sure how or why this occurs. Often, the child seems to control whether or not they throw up. It can be life-threatening, and a pediatrician must be consulted immediately to rule out organic or physical causes.

What should we eat before a race?

Eat normally. Special diets don't drastically boost performance. It is best to increase the amount of carbohydrates (pasta, cereals, beans) a few days before the race. Stay away from meat. Contrary to popular belief, eating meat does not boost performance and make you macho. Give yourselves about two to three hours digestion time before running. Drink plenty of water before and after the event.

What is your opinion of school lunches?

While we all seem to have our own story about some horrifying concoction we discovered in the school lunchroom, those meals are some of the best many American children eat. School lunches tend to be very well-balanced. Dieticians devise the menus to ensure that all food groups are represented. Overall, the nutrition, amount and price make it one of the best meal deals around.

There has been some recent controversy over excessive sugar and salt in some school district lunch programs. Find out what your school serves to know for sure if your child is getting good nutrition. See if all food groups are offered and what kinds of junk foods are available. Some parents forced school officials to remove vending machines when it was discovered that children were wasting lunch money on candy.

How many snacks per day?

Two to three. A snack is considered to be one serving from the various food groups. Children should have planned snacks throughout the day so they do not get too hungry. Snacks prevent overeating. Push fruit and vegetables. Try new exotic fruit as it arrives at your grocery store. Have vegetables cut and ready to eat in the refrigerator. Do not deprive your child of snacks. Let him eat as many fruits and vegetables as he wants.

If praise doesn't work all the time, then what?

TIME OUT. No, don't stop reading. I mean the child gets time out from rewards. This is an alternative to punishment. It works and does not have the emotional side effects of punishment.

When a child's behavior becomes sufficiently disruptive, say he pitches peas across the room, action must be taken. He is removed from the table and put in a place where he can't have fun. It must be a neutral room with no toys.

Sending him to the bedroom is not a good idea. That's where his playthings are. Instead, find a place that has little play value. A bathroom or laundry room will do well. *MAKE SURE NO OBJECTS, FLUIDS, CHEMICALS OR OTHER THINGS ARE AVAILABLE FOR THE CHILD TO HURT HIMSELF.*

Once an offense is committed, the child is banished to the Time Out room for five minutes. *Only five.* In order to return, he must wait for the time limit to be up. Then he can come back to the table.

Try to keep yourself as matter-of-fact as possible. Emotional upheaval will only prolong the bad behavior. If another offense occurs, a subsequent sentence of five minutes is handed down. The process is repeated as often as necessary.

Most children seek adult attention. By taking attention away via being alone, the bad behavior does not get reinforced. Bad behavior ceases to be rewarding. In order to be rewarded, good behavior must be displayed. When good behavior is shown, praise, praise and praise again.

One warning: Behavior gets worse before it gets better. If your child goes into wild contortions, that's OK. Be consistent. Put him in the room. At first he will protest loudly. In a few days, as hard as it may be for you to continue, you could be amazed at the change. Stick with it!

What is vomiting a sign of?

Possible trouble. Vomiting is a normal reflex that accompanies sickness. It is the body dumping matter suspected to be toxic. During an illness, it's normal. The stomach is irritated and ejects its contents. Alternately, prolonged vomiting can lead to dehydration. Dehydration can lead to severe complications if not corrected. If your child is vomiting heavily, go to your doctor immediately. He will be able to render a diagnosis and medicate if necessary.

Self-induced vomiting is a symptom of ANOREXIA NERVOSA and BULIMIA. It signals major psychological problems and needs professional help. If you suspect your child may be self-inducing vomiting, seek professional help from a psychologist or mental health worker who is trained in eating disorders. Don't delay.

Where To Go for Further Help

This program has brought you and your family some of the latest information on weight control. In mild to moderate situations, it can help greatly. It does take time, effort and awareness. Keep going. The long-term rewards for the whole family are well worth it.

At times, the family cannot treat itself. Self-help is a major undertaking that may not work for everyone. If you suspect your family's difficulties are beyond what you can change, understand that that situation is quite common. It takes a strong person to recognize the extent of his or her own limits and when to seek outside help. First, consult your physician. He can refer you to professionals who can offer help if he is unable to do so himself.

The next alternative in finding help is to contact your State Psychological Association or Medical Association. They have the names of professionals in your area who can help. Also, university departments of clinical psychology or psychiatry may support specialized programs that can assist you in your quest for family weight control. Go for a professional assessment if you have trouble meeting your goals. It is time well invested.

Final Word

Writing this book was a difficult but rewarding task. My only hope is that these pages bring to you and your family the knowledge that will help obtain weight control goals. Weight control is a difficult task, to be sure, but the rewards last a lifetime. *Everyone,* everywhere has to do it if he wishes to remain in optimal health. The average weight person has learned it naturally. So shall your children.

Most of all, you should have come to know that there are no free rides or magic pills for weight control. Consistent effort is necessary to obtain continuous good health and respectable bodyweight. Don't waste time and effort on fads, ads, or doodads. Change your habits. Nothing else will work on a long-term basis.

While weight control is healthy, a weight obsession is not. The whole family needs to realize that food is a part of life. It is something that powers the body—nothing more. People give it roles it can never completely fulfill. Don't fall into the same trap. Ultimately, you and your children can take control over the food in your lives. Don't let the *food* take control.

I sincerely wish the best to all of you. Live long and happy lives.

References

While not specifically cited in the text, the following dedicated scientists and their works contributed to the knowledge presented in this book.

American Alliance for Health, Physical Education, Recreation and Dance. *Health Related Physical Fitness Test Manual.* Reston, Va.: 1980.

American Coaching Effectiveness Program. Developed by Rainer Martins, Ph.D., University of Illinois, 1981.

Aragona, J., J. Cassidy, and R. Drabman. "Treating Overweight Children Through Parental Training and Contingency Contracting." *Journal of Applied Behavior Analysis* 8 (1975) 269–278.

Asher, A. "Fat Babies and Fat Children." *Archives of Diseases of Children* 41 (1966) 672.

Ashley, F. and W. Kannel. "Relation of Weight Change to Changes in Atherogenic Traits: The Framingham Study. *Journal of Chronic Diseases* 27 (1974) 103–114.

Bennett, G. "An Evaluation of Self-instructional Training in the Treatment of Obesity." *Addictive Behaviors* 11 (1986) 125–134.

Bjorntrop, P., L. Sjostrom and L. Sulivan. "The Role of Physical Exercise in the Management of Obesity." In *The Treatment of Obesity,* edited by J. Munroe. Lancaster, England: MTP Press, 1979.

Bloom, W. "Fasting as an Introduction to the Treatment of Obesity." *Metabolism* 8 (1959) 214.

Bray, G. *The Obese Patient.* Philadelphia: W. B. Saunders Co., 1976.

Broak, C., R. Huntly and J. Slack. "Influence of Heredity and Environment in Determination of Skinfold Thickness in Children." *British Medical Journal* 2 (1975) 719–721.

Brooks, C. "Evidence for a Sensitive Period in Adipose Cell Replication in Man." *Lancet* 11 (1973) 1036.

Brown, R. "Exercise and Mental Health in the Pediatric Population." *Clinical Sports Medicine* 1 (1982) 515–527.

Brownell, K. and A. Stunkard. "Behavioral Treatment for Obese Children and Adolescents." In *Obesity,* edited by A. Stunkard. Philadelphia: W. B. Saunders Co., 1980.

Bruch, H. "Obesity in Childhood: Physical Growth and Development of Obese Children." *American Journal of Diseases of Children* 8 (1939) 457–484.

Bruch, H. "Fat Children Grow Up." *American Journal of Diseases of Children* 90 (1955) 201.

Bruch, H. "Obesity in Childhood and Adolescence." *Postgraduate Medicine* 22 (1957) 146–151.

Bruch, H. *Eating Disorders.* New York: Basic Books, 1973.

Bruch, H. and G. Tourmaine. "Obesity in Childhood: The Family Frame of Obese Children." *Psychosomatic Medicine* 2 (1940) 141.

Burd, B. "Infant Swimming Classes: Immersed in Controversy." *The Physician and Sportsmedicine* 14 (1986) 239–244.

Caine, D. and K. Linder. "Growth Plate Injury: A Threat to Young Distance Runners?" *The Physician and Sportsmedicine* 12 (1986) 118–124.

Canning, H. and J. Mayer. "Obesity: Its Possible Effects on College Acceptance." *New England Journal of Medicine* 275 (1966) 1172–1174.

Coates, T. and C. Thoresen. Treating Obesity in Children and Adolescents: A Review." *American Journal of Public Health* 68 (1978) 143–151.

Cohen, E., D. Gelfand, D. Dodd and C. Turner. "Self-control Practices Associated with Weight Loss Maintenance in Children and Adolescents." *Behavior Therapy* 11 (1980) 26–37.

Committee on Nutrition, American Academy of Pediatrics. "Factors Affecting Food Intake." *Pediatrics* 33 (1964) 135.

Corbin, C. *A Textbook of Motor Development.* Dubuque, IA: William Brown Co., 1973.

Court, J. "Obesity in childhood." *Medical Journal of Austin* 1 (1977) 888–891.

Dauncey, M. and D. Gairdner. "Size of Adipose Cells in Infancy." *Archives of Diseases in Childhood* 50 (1975) 286–290.

Epstein, L., B. Masek and W. Marshall. "A Nutritionally Based School Program for Control of Eating in Obese Children." *Behavior Therapy* 9 (1978) 766–778.

Epstein, L., R. Wing, L. Steranchak, B. Dickson and J. Michelson. "Comparison of Family-based Behavior Modification and Nutrition Education for Childhood Obesity." *Journal of Pediatric Psychology* 5 (1980) 25–36.

Garn, S. and D. Clark. "Trends in Fatness and the Origins of Obesity." *Pediatrics* 57 (1976) 443–455.

Garrow, J. *Energy Balance and Obesity in Man.* New York: Elsevier, 1974.

Gold, D. "Psychological Factors Associated with Obesity." *American Family Physician* 13 (1979) 87–91.

Gorden, E. "Metabolic Aspects of Obesity." *Advanced Metabolic Disorders* 4 (1970) 229–296.

Gross, I., M. Wheeler and R. Hess. "The Treatment of Obesity in Adolescents Using Behavioral Self-control." *Clinical Pediatrics* 5 (1976) 920–924.

Hardcastle, D., L. Kerr and I. Smith. "Helping Obese School Girls to Lose Weight." *Connecticut Medicine* 128 (1972) 107.

Harris, M. and E. Hallbauer. "Self-directed Weight Control Through Eating and Exercise." *Behavior Therapy* 11 (1973) 523–529.

Hearld, F. and R. Hollander. "The Relationship Between Obesity in Adolescence and Early Growth." *Journal of Pediatrics* 51 (1965) 35.

Hirsh, J. "Can We Modify the Number of Adipose Cells?" *Post Graduate Medicine* 51 (1972) 83–86.

Hoffman, R. "Obesity in Childhood and Adolescence." *American Journal of Clinical Nutrition* 5 (1957) 1.

Jelliffe, D. *The Nutritional Status of the Community.* WHO Monograph, no. 53, WHO, 1966, 227.

Johnson, M., B. Burke, and J. Mayer. "The Prevalence and Incidence of Obesity in a Cross Section of Elementary and Secondary School Children." *American Journal of Clinical Nutrition* 4 (1956) 231.

Kannel, W. and T. Dawber. "Atherosclerosis as a Pediatric Problem." *Journal of Pediatrics* 80 (1972) 544–554.

Keane, T., S. Geller and C. Scherier. "A Parametric Investigation of Eating Styles in Obese and Non-obese Children." *Behavior Therapy* 12 (1981) 280–286.

Kingsley, R. and J. Shapiro. "A Comparison of Three Behavioral Programs for the Control of Obesity in Children." *Behavior Therapy* 8 (1977) 33–36.

Knittle, J. "Basic Concepts in the Control of Childhood Obesity." In *Childhood Obesity,* edited by M. Minichm. New York: John Wiley and Sons, 1975.

Krauses, M. and K. Mahon. *Food, Nutrition and Diet Therapy.* 6th ed. Philadelphia: W. B. Saunders Co., 1979.

Lloyd, J., O. Wolff and W. Whelen. "Childhood: A Long Term Study of Height and Weight." *British Medical Journal* 2 (1961) 651–660.

Marlina, R. "Exercise as an Influence Upon Growth." *Clinical Pediatrics* (1969) 16–26.

Marston, A., P. London and L. Cooper. "A Note on the Eating Behavior of Children Varying in Weight." *Journal of Child Psychology and Psychiatry* 17 (1976) 221–224.

Meichenbaum, D. *Cognitive-behavior Modification: An Integrative Approach.* New York: Plenum, 1977.

Meichenbaum, D. and J. Goodman. "Reflection-impulsivity and Verbal Control of Motor Behavior." *Child Development* 40 (1969) 785–797.

Meichenbaum, D. and J. Goodman. "Training Impulsive Children to Talk to Themselves: A Means of Developing Self-control." *Journal of Abnormal Psychology* 77 (1971) 115–126.

Morris, R. and T. Kratochwill, eds. *The Practice of Child Therapy.* New York: Pergamon Press, 1983.

Mullins, A. "The Prognosis of Juvenile Obesity." *Archives of Diseases of Childhood* 33 (1958) 307.

Neuman, C. "Obesity in the Pre-school and School Age Child." *Pediatric Clinics of North America* 24 (1977) 117–122.

Norsieck, A. "Relationship of Excess Weight in Children and Adults." *Public Health Report* 75 (1960) 263–273.

Powers, P. *Obesity: The Regulation of Weight.* Baltimore: Williams and Wilkins Co., 1980.

Raynor, P. "Effects of Dietary Restriction and Anoretic Drugs on Linear Growth in Childhood Obesity." *Archives of Diseases of Childhood* 49 (1974) 822.

Revinus, T., T. Drummond, and L. Combrinde-Graham. "A Group Behavior Treatment Program for Overweight Children: Results of a Pilot Study." *Pediatric and Adolescent Endocrinology* 1 (1976) 55–61.

Rowland, T. and P. Hoonis. "Organizing Road Races for Children: Special Concerns." *The Physician and Sportsmedicine* 13 (1985) 126–132.

Rose, H. and J. Mayer. "Activity, Caloric Intake and the Energy Balance of Infants." *Pediatrics* 41 (1968) 18–29.

Ryan, A. "The Very Young Athlete." *The Physician and Sportsmedicine* 11 (1983) 45.

Sallade, J. "A Comparison of the Psychological Adjustment of Obese and Non-obese Children." *Journal of Psychosomatic Residencies* 17 (1973) 89–96.

Sasaki, J., M. Shindo, and H. Tanaka, et al. "A Long-term Aerobic Exercise Program Decreases the Obesity Index and Increases the High Density Lipoprotein Cholesterol Concentration in Obese Children." *International Journal of Obesity* 11 (1987) 339–345.

Satter, E. "Childhood Eating Disorders." *Journal of the American Dietetic Association* 86 (1986) 357–361.

Satter, E. "The Feeding Relationship." *Journal of the American Dietetic Association* 86 (1986) 352.

Seigal, J. and T. Manfredi. "Effects of a Ten-month Fitness Program on Children." *The Physician and Sportsmedicine* 12 (1984) 91–97.

Speer, D. and K. Braun. "The Biochemical Basis of Growth Plate Injuries." *The Physician and Sportsmedicine* 13 (1986) 72–78.

Stuart, R. "Behavioral Control of Overeating." *Behavior Therapy* 5 (1967) 357–365.

Stunkard, A., E. D'Aquila, S. Fox, and D. Ross. "Influence of Social Class on Obesity and Thinness in Children." *Journal of the American Medical Association* 221 (1972) 597.

Sweeney, R., ed. *Selected Readings in Movement Education.* Addison-Wesley Publishing Co., 1970.

Tanner, J. and R. Whitehouse. "Standards for Subcutaneous Fat in British Children." *British Medical Journal* 446 (1962).

Tartz, L. "Infantile Overnutrition Among Artificially Fed Infants in the Sheffield Region." *British Journal of Medicine* 1 (1971) 315–316.

Tystad, O. "Childhood Obesity with Particular Reference to Etiological Factors." *World Medical Journal* 3 (1972) 45.

Tolstrup, K. "On Psychogenic Obesity in Children." *Acta Paediatrica* 42 (1953) 289–304.

Ward, A. "Born to Jog: Programs for Preschoolers." *The Physician and Sportsmedicine* 14 (1986) 163–167.

Waxman, M. and A. Stunkard. "Caloric Intake and Expenditure of Obese Boys." *Journal of Pediatrics* 96 (1980) 187–193.

Weinsier, R., et al. "Recommended Therapeutic Guidelines for Professional Weight Control Programs." *American Journal of Clinical Nutrition* 40 (1984) 865–872.

Wheeler, M. and K. Hess. "Treatment of Juvenile Obesity by Successive Approximation Control of Eating." *Journal of Behavior Therapy and Experimental Psychology* 7 (1976) 235–241.

Wilmore, J. and J. McNamara. "Prevalence of Coronary Heart Disease Risk Factors in Boys, 8 to 12 Years of Age." *Journal of Pediatrics* 84 (1974) 527–533.

Wolff, O. "Obesity in Childhood." *Quarterly Journal of Medicine* 24 (1955) 109.

Wood, D. "Aerobic Dance for Children: Resources and Recommendations." *The Physician and Sportsmedicine* 14 (1986) 225–229.

YMCA Division of Aquatics. *YMCA Guidelines for Infant Swimming*. Chicago: YMCA of the USA, 1984.

Zimmerman, B. and T. Rosenthal. "Observational Learning of Rule Governed Behavior in Children." *Psychological Bulletin* 81 (1974) 29–42.